Fortify Your LIFE

Also by Tieraona Low Dog

Healthy at Home
Life Is Your Best Medicine
(co-author) *National Geographic Guide to Medicinal Herbs*

Fortify Your LIFE

Your Guide to Vitamins, Minerals, and More

TIERAONA LOW DOG, M.D.

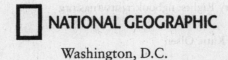

NATIONAL GEOGRAPHIC

Washington, D.C.

Published by the National Geographic Society
1145 17th Street N.W., Washington, D.C. 20036

Library of Congress Cataloging-in-Publication Data
ISBN 978-1-4262-1668-8

The National Geographic Society is one of the world's largest nonprofit
scientific and educational organizations. Its mission is to inspire people to
care about the planet. Founded in 1888, the Society is member supported
and offers a community for members to get closer to explorers, connect with
other members, and help make a difference. The Society reaches more than
450 million people worldwide each month through *National Geographic*
and other magazines; National Geographic Channel; television documen-
taries; music; radio; films; books; DVDs; maps; exhibitions; live events;
school publishing programs; interactive media; and merchandise. National
Geographic has funded more than 10,000 scientific research, conservation,
and exploration projects and supports an education program promoting geographic literacy. For more information, visit www.nationalgeographic.com.

National Geographic Society
1145 17th Street N.W.
Washington, D.C. 20036-4688 U.S.A.

For information about special discounts for bulk purchases, please contact
National Geographic Books Special Sales: ngspecsales@ngs.org

For rights or permissions inquiries, please contact National Geographic
Books Subsidiary Rights: ngbookrights@ngs.org

Interior design: Katie Olsen

16/xxx/1 [Product code, TK from Managing Ed. once printer is awarded]

To Richard and Vivian,
with deep gratitude and love for the life I was given

Disclaimer

This book is designed as a reference volume and is made available to the public with the understanding that the author and the publisher are not rendering medical or other professional advice tailored to individual needs and situations. You should not use the information contained in this book as a substitute for the advice of a licensed health-care professional and should consult a health-care professional to address any health concerns specific to you.

Because nutritional supplements can interact with medications or affect some medical conditions, you should always check with your prescribing health-care professional before using the herbal remedies described in this book.

The author and publisher disclaim any liability whatsoever with respect to any loss, injury, or damage arising out of the use of the information contained in this book or omission from any information in this book.

Mention of specific products, companies, or organizations does not imply that the publisher and author of this book endorse such products, companies, or organizations.

Contents

Preface   XX

Introduction   XX

CHAPTER 1: Life Fortified   XX

CHAPTER 2: Inside the Bottle and Behind the Label   XX

CHAPTER 3: Vitamins   XX

CHAPTER 4: Minerals   XX

CHAPTER 5: Nutraceuticals   XX

CHAPTER 6: Supplements for Common Ailments   XX

CHAPTER 7: Making Sense of Health Information   XX

APPENDIX 1: Your Food Journal   XX

APPENDIX 2: Your Personalized Supplements Chart   XX

APPENDIX 3: Laboratory Tests   XX

APPENDIX 4: Drug-Nutrient Depletions and Interactions   XX

Glossary   XX

Contents

Preface xx

Introduction xx

CHAPTER 1: The Fortified xx

CHAPTER 2: Inside the Bottle and Behind the Label xx

CHAPTER 3: Vitamins xx

CHAPTER 4: Minerals xx

CHAPTER 5: Nutraceuticals xx

CHAPTER 6: Supplements for Common Ailments xx

CHAPTER 7: Making Sense of Health Information xx

APPENDIX 1: Your Food Journal xx

APPENDIX 2: Your Personalized Supplement Chart xx

APPENDIX 3: Laboratory Tests xx

APPENDIX 4: Drug-Nutrient Depletions and Interactions xx

Glossary xx

Preface

I awoke to the phone ringing at 11 p.m. I thought to myself, "Nothing good ever comes from a phone call late at night." It was my mother. My father had been admitted to the hospital. She couldn't really explain what had happened, just that "some of his numbers" were off. I called my dad's cell phone and when I heard his voice, I was taken aback by how weak he sounded. He's in relatively good health despite being 80 years old and having had cancer for many, many years. But he had taught school for most of this past year and was quite active: a testament to his inner strength and healthy outlook on life. Other than the medication he takes every three months for his cancer, my father only takes a proton pump inhibitor (PPI) that he's been on for many years; a mild diuretic for his blood pressure; and a small assortment of supplements: magnesium, fish oil, calcium, and vitamin D. Roughly two weeks before he was admitted to the hospital, he started having diarrhea. He didn't think much about it, other than it was annoying when he was at school. Then he started to feel weak and his legs began to cramp. One morning he just couldn't get up out of bed. My mom took him to the urgent care clinic.

I asked what the doctors had told him. "Well, honey, it seems that my potassium and magnesium are low, dangerously low, too low to go home. They want to tank me up before they let me go." The doctors gave him intravenous fluids to deliver these two vital nutrients and sent him home after 24 hours. One week later he was back in the hospital, his levels low again. This time I insisted on speaking with someone on his medical team.

Proton pump inhibitors can cause lots of problems when you take them a long time. They are notorious for robbing the body of key nutrients, such as magnesium, calcium, and vitamins B12 and D. And they increase the risk for both pneumonia and an intestinal infection known as *Clostridium difficile*, or *C. diff.* This time, the doctor ordered a stool culture to see what was causing his diarrhea and, sure enough, my father had *C. diff.*, a nasty bug that can sometimes be very hard to treat. Dad had assured me that every three months his labs were getting drawn and that everything was normal. But when I asked, there was no record of a magnesium level having been recently checked. The PPI had caused him to have diarrhea, which in combination with his diuretic drug, tipped his already precarious magnesium level to a life-threatening level. His potassium was dangerously low, as well. Talking to the physician and hearing just how low my father's electrolytes were, I was in shock and disbelief. He could easily have died.

This story is just one of many examples of the unintended consequences of doctors prescribing multiple drugs to a patient, as well as the unique challenges of caring for elders who do not have the same vital reserves as someone 40 or 50 years younger. We are going to see more and more problems as baby boomers age and have multiple medical conditions, take multiple prescription medications, see numerous doctors, and have no one coordinating their care.

I've had to toe to toe with some of his doctors over these past 20 years. One told him he didn't need a bone density scan to screen for osteoporosis or his vitamin D level checked, despite the fact that he had become several inches shorter and routinely complained of back and hip pain. Yes, he had osteoporosis and his vitamin D level was low. My father was also told he didn't need to have his B12 level checked, even though my mother told me that he was feeling increasingly depressed and fatigued. His doctor said to me, "Your father has stage 4 cancer and is 74 years old. Don't you think that could be why he's feeling depressed and tired?" I wanted to scream. When Dad went on chemo in 2009, he was put on a PPI. A year later I suggested that he try to wean off it but his physician recommended he stay on it. He also reassured my father that he could get all the nutrients he needed by just eating a good diet. And yet, not once did the physician *ever* even ask my father what he eats or refer him to a dietitian.

To say that I have felt frustrated with my father's care over the years would be an understatement. On the one hand, I am so very grateful that his team of providers has kept his cancer under control so that he could still be in our lives, for I love my father more than words could ever express. On the other hand, I wish that the conversations had been broad enough to encompass a wide range of topics that could have improved my father's quality of life. While it is hard to admit, the fact is that nutrition and nutritional supplements are so far off the radar that more than a few professionals in mainstream medicine made me feel like some sort of quack for just asking questions about my father's nutritional needs.

I am a medical doctor, but I am also a daughter, wife, mother, and cancer patient. I believe that a knowledgeable patient is an empowered patient. We have to take charge of our own health and try to find skilled and compassionate practitioners along the way who are open to taking the journey with us. I wrote this book to help you navigate the complex and often confusing landscape of nutritional supplements. This will not be the only book or resource you need, however. I did not write an exhaustive list of every supplement product in the marketplace: There are more than 30,000! Instead, I chose to focus on the foundation of nutrition: the building blocks in food that are necessary for your body to carry out the thousands of biochemical jobs it must perform every single day. While that new berry from the Amazonian jungle may indeed be a miracle, you won't find information about it in this book. I'd prefer you truly understand why your body needs thiamine, pyridoxine, and zinc and what happens when you are lacking in any of them. I want you to think about what nutrients are responsible for making the brain chemicals responsible for mood before you simply reach for the St. John's wort or, for that matter, the Prozac. If you started taking the medication captopril for your blood pressure and now three months later you're experiencing some loss of taste, I want you to realize it's due to the loss of zinc. I want you to know which of the many commonly prescribed drugs can rob your body of precious life-generating nutrients and what you can do to prevent your levels of them from falling so low you end up in the hospital.

My father's case is far more common than you could ever imagine. It is because of him, and the thousands of people who have shared their lives and their stories with me, that I wrote this book. I hope it will be of value to you.

Introduction

I was older than most prospective doctors are when I went to medical school. I'd already studied massage therapy, martial arts, and midwifery and had opened and run my own herb company. I was excited when I finished meeting all the undergraduate requirements and was accepted to the University of New Mexico School of Medicine in Albuquerque. It was a phenomenal school with amazing teachers. I learned a great many things, but in four years of medical school education, we maybe spent three to five hours on nutrition and virtually none on nutritional supplements. The discussion on nutrition was principally around a case involving a 60-year-old patient who showed up in the emergency room complaining of confusion and difficulty walking. As students, our job was to work through all the different possibilities of what could be causing her symptoms, figure out what testing would be necessary to come up with a diagnosis, and then recommend the optimal treatment. The lesson was designed to teach us about Wernicke's encephalopathy, a nasty brain disorder caused by a lack of vitamin B1 (thiamine) that can cause confusion, uncontrolled eye movements, difficulty walking, loss of memory, and in severe cases, coma and death. It primarily occurs in alcoholics although it can also occur in others who are malnourished due to diet, persistent vomiting, or disease. Tragically, on my neurology rotation during my family practice internship, we admitted a patient very much like the case I'd studied as a student.

But other than a few references here and there to very serious nutritional deficiencies, my fellow students and I had no in-depth training on nutrition or nutritional supplements. I learned to read an EKG and diagnose heart disease, but not how to counsel these patients on the key components of a heart-healthy diet. I was prescribing multiple cardiovascular medications, but no attending physician taught me to monitor anything other than sodium and potassium when my patients were on these drugs. As for our pregnant or breastfeeding mothers, we were only taught to give the most basic nutritional guidance on folic acid, calcium, and avoiding alcohol and smoking.

When I reflect upon my own training, it's easy for me to understand why physicians often overlook nutrition and nutritional supplements. Most of us went into clinical practice thinking that the vast majority of people get what they need from the food they eat and that when something goes wrong in the body, it can usually be fixed with medication or surgery. I don't think physicians are alone in this thinking. I bet many Americans also believe that they're getting everything they need in their diet. You may even believe it. I don't.

For the past 20 years I've been asking patients to fill out a two- to three-day food journal to see what they are actually eating so I can better see whether there are any nutritional gaps. They might start their day with sugary breakfast cereal accompanied by two cups of coffee; then a sandwich with lunchmeat on white bread with mustard, along with a cookie and a soda for lunch; and finish up with a burger with fries and more soda for dinner.

The closest thing to dark leafy green vegetables was the little bit of iceberg lettuce on their fast-food hamburger.

My experience consistently shows me that a large number of Americans live high-carb, high-sugar, caffeine-overloaded, stressed-out, no-exercise lives. We may have good intentions when it comes to eating well, but the truth is that most of us fall far short of an ideal diet.

It wasn't that long ago in the United States—in some cases less than 100 years ago—that we saw the disastrous consequences of nutritional deficiencies. In later chapters we'll talk about rickets, scurvy, goiter, and pellagra, which are rarely seen nowadays but were a big problem for earlier generations. However, we are beginning to see some nutrient deficiencies on the rise again. It was because of goiter that the Morton Salt Company starting putting iodine in table salt in 1924. After being an "iodine sufficient" nation for more than half a century, we are once again starting to see low iodine levels. This is the result of public health messages to cut back on salt, the fact that the salt found in processed food and fast food does not contain iodine, and more people are using non-iodized specialty salts. The U.S. government mandated the enrichment of grains with thiamine (vitamin B1), riboflavin (vitamin B2), niacin (vitamin B3), folic acid (vitamin B9), and iron. Yet many people are starting to avoid grains because of concerns over gluten sensitivity and celiac disease, which makes them vulnerable to vitamin B deficiencies. And many of the foods and cereals being certified non-GMO (non–genetically modified organisms) are not enriched with any additional vitamins, as the companies cannot guarantee with certainty that the vitamins came from a non-GMO source. Sorting through all this information isn't easy and trying to figure out what *you* need isn't always straightforward.

In an attempt to make nutrition easier to understand, national guidelines have been created to tell us how much protein, fat, fiber, vitamins, minerals, and other nutrients we should be getting on a daily basis. These dietary recommendations vary based upon your age, gender, and whether you are pregnant or breastfeeding. Using information from the United States Department of Agriculture (USDA), the Food and Drug Administration (FDA), and the National Academy of Medicine (NAM, until recently named the Institute of Medicine, or IOM), I've calculated how much of a particular food you'd have to eat to get either the daily value (DV) or recommended daily allowance (RDA) for some of the key vitamins and minerals.

Are you ready? You might be surprised by some of these numbers.

Vitamin B6 (1.5 mg):
2.5 bananas
12 Tbsp. roasted sunflower seeds
8 ounces chicken breast
5 ounces beef liver
12–13 ounces tuna, light canned
3.75 cups cooked lentils
3.5 cups raw diced avocado
20 Tbsp. peanut butter

Vitamin B12 (6 mcg):
1 small clam
0.2 ounces beef liver
2.3 ounces canned sardines
7–8 ounces ground beef
7–8 large eggs
6 cups almond or soy milk
5 cups yogurt
6.4 ounces Atlantic salmon

Vitamin D (600 IU):
3.5–4 ounces sockeye salmon, cooked

11.4 ounces water-packed tuna
26 oil-packed sardines
15 large eggs
5 cups fortified milk
45 ounces yogurt

Vitamin E (30 IU/20 mg):
5.4 Tbsp. roasted sunflower seeds
3.6 Tbsp. sunflower seed oil
5 Tbsp. almond butter
13.2 ounces light or firm tofu
4–5 cups cooked spinach
5 cups canned tomato sauce
18–20 large eggs, cooked

Iron (18 mg):
4.5 cups raisins
3–5 cups instant oatmeal
2.2 cups canned white beans
10 ounces beef liver
3 cups Special K cereal
45 ounces chicken breast
3 cups cooked lentils
15 cups broccoli
3 cups cooked spinach

Magnesium (400 mg):
2.5 cups boiled spinach
2.5 cups Swiss chard
6.5 cups soy milk
9 ounces tofu
17 slices whole wheat bread
3.5 cups cooked black beans
2.5 cups pumpkin seeds
4.7 cups cooked brown rice

Kind of shocking isn't it? Some foods, such as sardines, clams, oysters, and beef liver, are nutrient powerhouses but not standard fare at most dinner tables. Salmon or tuna are excellent dietary sources of vitamins B12 and D, and omega-3 fatty acids, but because of mercury levels, we're limited to no more than 4 ounces two to three times per week. Agricultural scientists have shown that the nutritional value of our fruits and vegetables has declined, in some cases significantly, over the past 40 years. We are exposed to more and more environmental toxins that strain our body's defense systems, and half of all Americans take at least one prescription drug, many of which further deplete the body's vital nutrients. It's difficult to get all the nutrients we need on a regular basis with diet alone—not impossible, but hard.

If, like most people, you're trying but failing to eat a great diet, or if you have a specific medical condition, take prescriptions medications, are planning on becoming or are pregnant or nursing, are an athlete, are over the age of 50, or just want to enhance your health—I believe a basic multivitamin-mineral supplement, as well as a few other strategically chosen nutritional supplements, such as probiotics, omega-3 fatty acids, and possibly additional magnesium and vitamin D, could make a big difference in helping you achieve your health goals, while reducing your risk for chronic disease and supporting a healthy mood, body, and energy level.

I always ask my patients to bring all their supplements with them to their appointments. It's not an exaggeration to say that many arrive with a bagful of bottles. When I take each bottle out and ask why they are taking it, many are unable to tell me why. They read somewhere that a particular nutrient is "good for you," or heard on a television show that it prevents or treats this or that. They frequently admit they're not sure whether the supplement is working for them, or how much they should be taking. When I dive deeper into their food and lifestyle choices, it becomes clear that many are uncertain how to wade through the flood of health information out there to discern what is important for *them*. I'm sympathetic. How do we make sense of all the information and manufacturers' claims that are out there? How do we separate the truth from the hype? And what does it really mean to each of us personally?

We live in an age of information—you can take out your smartphone right now and access endless amounts of information on nutritional supplements. But the question is: Do you know what to *do* with that information? Does it help you make personalized choices about *your* health? Or does it leave you feeling overwhelmed and unsure of whether you're getting what your body needs without overdoing it?

Contradictory information about nutrition is everywhere. One day you'll hear that a daily multivitamin-mineral supplement "doesn't do anything" and "isn't necessary if you're eating well," and the next, you'll hear that few Americans are getting enough vitamin D or magnesium in their diet. If we aren't supposed to take supplements, and we aren't getting these key nutrients in our diet, where exactly are we supposed to get them? Different government websites provide conflicting nutritional information and advice. If you're like many busy people, you don't have the time or the expertise to figure out what all the nutrition information out there means for you or your family members.

Every year, I travel the country and teach thousands of lay people as well as physicians and other health-care professionals about the appropriate use of nutritional supplements. Pharmaceutical drugs are a gift, but are not always the best option. With high health-care costs, an aging population, and the growing burden of heart disease, diabetes, cancer, and other health challenges facing us all, we are overdue for learning how to take better care for ourselves. Lifestyle choices and managing stress are vital to our well-being, which is why I wrote an entire book about taking charge of your health: *Life Is Your Best Medicine*. My next book, *Healthy at Home,* was written to help you recognize when you could use simple, natural interventions for common minor ailments and when you should go see your health-care provider.

I have always believed that nutritional supplements can be an important adjunct to a healthy lifestyle. It is time for a broader, rational discussion on the topic of supplements that goes beyond the confusing sound bites and outdated, fragmented, distorted information about vitamins, minerals, and other important nutrients that the media is bombarding us with today. I wrote this book because I want to help you make informed decisions about the foundational supplements that are necessary for the life and times in which you are living. I want you to know how to choose the right supplements and work with your health-care providers to foster the best possible health—for *you.*

HOW TO USE THIS BOOK

Fortify Your Life offers a personalized approach to using supplements because no one has the same exact nutritional needs that you do. Whatever the condition of your health, whatever your lifestyle choices are, be aware that supplements should always be seen as just that, a *supplement* for good health practices, not a *substitute* for them. You can't live on highly processed foods, never exercise, or allow your anxiety and emotional stress to spin out of control, and then expect supplements to be the magic fix for the health problems you will surely develop from a lifetime of poor choices and poor health management. That would be like driving a car while texting and drunk, in the dark with your headlights off, in oncoming traffic, and expecting your seatbelt to keep you safe. No seatbelt can make up for that disastrous set of circumstances! However, I believe that if you make a genuine effort to eat well; manage stress; get the quality rest you need; exercise; and maintain healthy relationships with family, friends, and people in your community (yes, all of that contributes to good health), then just like a seatbelt, nutritional supplements can add an extra layer of protection.

In this book, you will learn the basics about the foundational supplements: vitamins, minerals, omega-3 fatty acids, probiotics, choline, and a small handful of others; which ones are necessary on a daily basis and which ones you might want to consider if you have certain health conditions or are at a particular stage of your life, such as preparing to become pregnant or are entering your elder years. In Chapters 1 and 2, I'll introduce the most important ideas for understanding supplements and how they work, and explain why personalizing your approach is important. In Chapters 3 and 4, you'll learn about the most important supplements—the vitamins and minerals your body needs on a regular basis, and how to make sense of the various forms seen in the marketplace. Chapter 5 will cover a few of the most important non–vitamin and mineral supplements, or nutraceuticals (a catchall term for nutritional supplements that are not vitamins, minerals, or herbal remedies) that you might want to take depending on your unique health profile and how these supplements interact with the biochemistry of your body. In Chapter 6, you'll learn about what supplements you should consider based upon your lifestyle, age, gender and if you have a certain health condition. In Chapter 7, you'll learn how to make sense of research and health reporting, and receive guidance on teaming with physicians and other professionals who may not be as informed about nutrition as they should be.

In the back of this book, you will find helpful information for creating your own personalized plan for using nutritional supplements for health, wellness, and vitality. You'll find a form for creating a food journal, as well as charts for noting the best times of the day for taking supplements and identifying possible drug-nutrient interactions and drug-induced nutrient depletions, and resources for further educating yourself on what you can do to improve or maintain your health.

All of us are busy these days, trying to keep up with the demands of our lives while sifting through all the information coming at us from every direction. My hope is that this book will make sorting out important health information easier for you, and leave you with the knowledge of how to choose and use nutritional supplements to achieve your personal wellness goals.

Chapter 1

Life Fortified

It was in the deep winter of 1535–36 in what is now Quebec City, Canada, that the crew of the French explorer Jacques Cartier developed scurvy. Dom Agaya, son of the Iroquois chief Donnacona, showed Cartier how to prepare a tea from the branches of the cedar tree that could treat the disease. The tea was so effective that Cartier proclaimed it a miracle that so many of his men survived. Is it any surprise then that the northern white cedar became known as the "tree of life?" Cedar needles were not part of the typical diet, but they were consumed during the long winters by indigenous peoples. In 1932, scientists finally determined that a lack of vitamin C is what causes scurvy. And guess what? Cedar needles contain vitamin C.

Many cultures around the world looked to nature for substances that could enhance their health during different seasons of the year as well as during different stages of their lives. In Traditional Chinese Medicine, physicians recommended medicinal plants to fortify the mind and body. Reishi, a nonculinary mushroom, was dried and consumed as tea to encourage vigor and long life. Scientists have found that reishi is a powerhouse antioxidant, helping protect the body from environmental toxins as well as shutting down excessive inflammation, which we know drives many chronic diseases. In Ayurveda, the traditional medicine of India, one category of plants, the rasayanas, were believed to promote health, protect the mind and memory, and support the body's ability to defend itself against infection and many of the degenerative processes that can happen as we age. Researchers are now finding that some of these rasayanas, such as bacopa, ashwagandha, and shatavari, have incredible promise for their ability to squelch inflammation and oxidative stress, as well as to support immune and brain health. So, when I hear the argument that people haven't traditionally "supplemented" their diet, I beg to differ. The concept of enhancing our health through supplementation is quite ancient. In my opinion, with all the stressors of modern life, we may need to fortify our lives more than ever before.

HOW OUR LIVES HAVE CHANGED

Modern advances in sanitation, public health initiatives, immunizations, and medicine have led to a dramatic decline in many acute and infectious diseases. My grandmother's brother died at age 13 in southwestern Kansas from a ruptured appendix because there were no local surgeons or hospitals. This was not uncommon just a few generations ago but is thankfully a rarity in the U.S. today. Early detection has allowed us to identify potentially life-threatening diseases early enough to successfully intervene in the disease process. There is so much to be thankful for when it comes to modern medicine. Yet, even with all these incredible advances, and there have been many, Americans are still faced with a staggering burden of chronic disease.

Almost one in ten people have diabetes and that number is rapidly growing. A disease once only seen in the elder population, type 2 diabetes now affects children as young as four years of age. Heart disease continues to be the number one cause of death for both men and women, with more than 70 percent of American adults taking medications to treat it in 2012. Dementia, or what was once called senility, is now diagnosed every 67 seconds in the U.S. And while researchers and clinicians work tirelessly to find the most effective ways to treat cancer, this devastating disease is on the rise in the young and old around the globe. Some experts believe that today's children will be the first generation in history to not live as long as their parents.

What is driving the rise in chronic disease? The answer is complex, as there are many factors at play. Diet, obesity, lack of physical activity, poor management of stress, inadequate rest and sleep, and exposure to environmental toxins are among the primary drivers of many of the chronic diseases plaguing 21st-century America. Our lives have changed dramatically over the past 100 years.

Our modern diet looks very different than that of our ancestors. People lived on wild game or meat—including organ meats and eggs sourced from their own livestock, as well as vegetables and fruits that were often grown in their own garden, along with legumes, nuts, and seeds. Depending upon where people lived, cheese, butter and whole grains were also consumed. But nowhere on the planet were people eating Pop-Tarts for breakfast or processed salty snack chips and soda pop for lunch. Processed foods are almost always lower in important nutrients than foods closer to their natural, whole form and they often contain substances, such as high-fructose corn syrup and artificial flavorings/colorings, which are foreign to our body. In the span of just 100 years, we've gone from roughly 8 pounds of added sugar per person per year to more than 100 pounds! More than one-third of this sugar comes from soda or energy and sports drinks, none of which were present in your great-grandmother's kitchen.

Plant-based foods are incredibly important for our health, and we require an abundance of them in our diet. With all the stresses of modern life, we need the antioxidants (substances that maintain cellular integrity and prevent damage do DNA) and phytonutrients (plant nutrients) found in fruits, vegetables, nuts, and seeds. However, in spite of public health messages encouraging us to eat 4 to 5 *cups* of vegetables and fruits every day, the average American falls far short. And when you read the latest news report touting an increase in vegetable intake, check the fine print. Two-thirds of this increase is generally attributed to potatoes, potato chips, and French fries—hardly the rich, rainbow-colored produce those who care about public health were hoping for!

And even if you are eating your fruits and veggies, their nutritional value has also changed. While modern agricultural advances have allowed farmers to grow larger varieties and quantities of produce, enabling us to feed the growing populations of the world, unfortunately, that bountiful harvest has come at a cost. Breeding plants for size, quick growth, long-distance transport, and weeks-long storage has made our veggies and fruits less nutritious. A landmark study published by Donald Davis et al., in the *Journal of the American College of Nutrition* in 2004, compared USDA nutrient data for 43 garden crops from 1950 to 1999. It found a statistically reliable decline in six important nutrients: a 6 percent decline in protein and a 15 to 38 percent decline in calcium, iron, riboflavin, phosphorous, and vitamin C.

And reduced nutrition in produce is not just a U.S. problem. A 2005 report from the United Kingdom noted that the average concentrations of copper, magnesium, and sodium in vegetables and copper, iron, and potassium in fruits decreased significantly between the 1930s and the 1980s. Another study of 20 commonly eaten vegetables published in the *British Food Journal* found that the average calcium content had declined 19 percent, iron by 22 percent, and potassium by 14 percent. With so many people in the world deficient in important vitamins and minerals, the declining concentration of almost half of all the essential nutrients in our produce is concerning.

It's not just the change in nutritional value that is alarming, but also the reality that the use of pesticides and herbicides is now common practice in farming. I recognize that there have been benefits associated with their use, but we can't ignore the damaging effects they can have on our health, particularly during pregnancy and childhood, when chemical exposures are most dangerous. Studies published in highly prestigious scientific/medical journals show that pesticides exposures, in utero and during childhood, may increase the risk of childhood leukemia and other childhood cancers, early female puberty, irregularities in menstrual and ovarian function, and attention-deficit-hyperactive disorder (ADHD). Long-term exposures, small "doses" over decades, can have a cumulative effect that may make us more vulnerable to prostate cancer, early menopause, breast cancer, and neurological harm. Certain toxic chemicals, such as PCBs, DDT, and dioxins, are classified as persistent organic pollutants because they persist in the environment for a very long-time. Although they have been banned, these chemicals that are known to adversely effect human health, continue to show up in our bones and bloodstream.

I believe that now more than ever, our cells need protection from the damaging effects of environmental pollutants. Studies show that vitamins A, C, and E, and melatonin (a hormone produced in the pineal gland) protect our body from organophosphate pesticides, dioxins, and PCBs. Yet, according to the Office of Dietary Supplements, most Americans don't meet the RDA for vitamin E from their diet alone—and melatonin, which plays a vital role in regulating our 24-hour circadian clock, is routinely suppressed by the constant exposure to blue light from computer screens, televisions, and house lights. Vitamins C and E also protect us against cigarette smoke, air pollution, and ultraviolet radiation. Yet 16 million Americans are severely deficient in vitamin C. Iron helps protect against lead toxicity, which is incredibly dangerous to the brain and nervous system of infants and young children. Yet seven percent of American children between the ages of one and five have iron deficiency anemia, and that number doubles among Hispanic children. The point is this: We are exposed to an increasing number and amount of chemicals in our food and environment and the typical American diet is not sufficient to protect our DNA and health from these toxins.

Our work lives have also changed: Many of us no longer spend much of our time outdoors as people did in centuries past. We live, work, and even play indoors. However, getting adequate exposure to sunlight is critical for maintaining a normal sleep-wake cycle, fostering healthy mood, and synthesizing vitamin D. And when we do go outside, we wear sunscreen. Most women, and many men, put on skin moisturizer every morning that contains an SPF of 15 or higher.

I'm not recommending that you get rid of your sunscreen. It's important to protect your skin from sun damage and reduce your risk for skin cancer. However, since sunscreen limits sun absorption, it also significantly limits the subsequent manufacture of vitamin D. It's very hard to get adequate amounts of vitamin D in the diet; the body was designed to produce it in the skin after exposure to sunlight. Vitamin D is not only vitally important for healthy bones; research shows that it also plays a significant role in immune and cardiovascular health. Vitamin D deficiency/ insufficiency among Americans is a big problem, particularly for those who are dark-skinned, spend most of their time indoors, regularly use sunscreen, live in northern latitudes, and/or who are overweight or obese. According to the Centers for Disease Control (CDC), at least 66 million Americans have low levels of vitamin D. Are you one of them?

Another change: our consumption of salt, as I mentioned earlier. In the early 20th century, goiter, a swelling of the thyroid gland, was common in areas around the Great Lakes and in the Pacific Northwest. When it was found that iodine could both treat and prevent goiter (iodine is critical for maintaining thyroid function), the Morton Salt Company began selling iodized salt in 1924. Salt was a perfect delivery system, as iodine didn't alter its taste, and both rich and poor consumed it regularly. Goiter was all but eradicated. Today, public health messages warn that excessive salt can increase blood pressure and harm the kidneys and cardiovascular system, so we've cut back, especially at home. And when we do use table salt, an increasing number of us are choosing from a variety of options now available in the marketplace: Himalayan, kosher, and sea salt. Unless they specifically say they are iodized, these salts are naturally very low in iodine. Fast foods and processed foods may be high in sodium but they don't contain iodized salt.

What's more, the chemical perchlorate, which is both naturally occurring and man-made, blocks the uptake of iodine by the thyroid gland. The Department of Defense and the National Aeronautics and Space Administration (NASA) use significant amounts of manufactured perchlorate in the production of rockets, munitions (grenades, flares, fuses), and missiles. The perchlorate can then contaminate groundwater and soil, making its way into our food and drinking water. Having lived in New Mexico much of my life, I'm very aware of this situation, given that two of our large military bases in southern New Mexico—Holloman Air Force Base and White Sands Missile Range—have been found to have, and continue to have, very high levels of perchlorate in both surface and ground water. Having adequate amounts of iodine in the diet is extremely important as it competes with perchlorate for binding sites on the thyroid, reducing some of the chemical's adverse effects.

Although the United States has been considered "iodine sufficient" for decades, the most recent large government nutrition study found that reproductive age women in this country are now borderline iodine insufficient. Canada reported similar findings. This is very troubling given that low iodine during pregnancy reduces IQ and increases the risk for impaired cognitive development in babies. A Mount Sinai study published in the *Journal of Women's Health* in 2014 found that 38.9 percent of the pregnant women attending prenatal clinics in New York City who were not taking iodine supplements were at risk for mild-to-severe iodine deficiency according to World Health Organization guidelines. The RDA for iodine is 150 to 290 micrograms (mcg) for adults and the American Thyroid Association now recommends that *all* pregnant and nursing women take a daily vitamin that provides 150 mcg of iodine as potassium iodide. This is one example of how dangerous it can be to dismiss supplements out of hand.

Another factor to consider: We take lots of prescription drugs. In fact, the U.S. population takes more medications than any other country on the planet. In 2011, Americans spent $263 billion on prescription drugs, accounting for almost 10 percent of all national health expenditures. According to the CDC report *Health: United States 2013,* about 50 percent of Americans take at least one prescription drug per day and 10 percent take five or more. You may need to take a pharmaceutical drug for months or years, but do you know the effects of that drug on your body's ability to absorb and use key nutrients in your diet?

Proton pump inhibitors, or PPIs (drugs that inhibit the proton, or acid-producing, pumps in the stomach) are one of the most widely prescribed classes of drugs in the U.S. Sold under such brand names as Nexium, Prilosec, and Protonix, they are used to treat acid reflux—and are, in my opinion, overprescribed. Stomach acid is vitally important for your ability to absorb and/or utilize many key nutrients, including iron, calcium, magnesium and vitamin B12. PPIs carry an FDA black box warning that they can increase your risk for bone fracture and cause your magnesium levels to drop dangerously low, increasing the risk for seizures and serious heart arrhythmias. Most physicians are not aware of, nor do they monitor for, these potentially severe nutritional depletions. And there are many such nutrient-depleting medications. Metformin, a frequently prescribed drug for diabetes causes B12 deficiency, especially if you take it for more than four years. ACE inhibitors and thiazide diuretics used to treat high blood pressure deplete zinc. The list goes on and on. Many patients taking these drugs have never been checked for specific nutrient deficiencies and no clinician has told them to either increase their dietary intake of foods rich in these vitamins/minerals, take a supplement, or both.

If you look closely at the multitude of ways that our lives, diets, foods, and medication use have changed over the past 100 years, it becomes clear that there may be gaps in your nutrition, as well as higher needs for certain nutrients based upon your age, gender, personal health history, use of medications, and level of exposure to environmental toxins and other stressors.

WHY SUPPLEMENTS MATTER

I hope you're beginning to see that your diet may not be enough to ensure that you are getting all the key nutrients necessary for life in the 21st century. Fortunately, we can draw upon a large body of research on nutrition and nutritional supplements to help us in our pursuit of better health. A quick search of the National Library of Medicine online resource PubMed yields more than 307,000 citations on nutrition, 535,000 on micronutrients, 33,000 for the combination of calcium and health, 44,000 for vitamin D and health, and 23,000 articles just on iron deficiency. However, with the rate of medical knowledge doubling every three years, and expected to double every 73 days by the year 2020, clearly, it's impossible for any clinician to keep up with all the data. This is why it is important that *you* learn how to take charge of your own health, so that you can make informed decisions for you and your family.

It can be hard to sort through the noise. If you have a particular illness or disease, you've probably already started researching what nutritional support may be beneficial for you. But even if you're generally healthy, it's still important to be aware that low levels of key nutrients can significantly stress your body. That is why I want to help you recognize your risks for being deficient in certain nutrients, figure out what nutritional supplements might help you address those deficiencies, and know what to look for when purchasing nutritional supplements for yourself and your loved ones.

You want to make sure you fasten your seatbelt when it comes to nutrition and, when appropriate, take the supplements that offer the most protection. If you have a chronic health problem, you might be surprised by how much better you feel when you choose the correct nutritional and supplement regimen. You might even be able to slow the progression of your disease. You can feel confident that you are supporting your health by optimizing your nutrition—without wasting money or taking dozens of capsules or tablets each day.

Chapter 2

Inside the Bottle and Behind the Label

When I was the fellowship director at the University of Arizona Center for Integrative Medicine, I took groups of physicians and nurse practitioners to the local natural foods grocery, where I gave them notecards containing short vignettes of patients with particular health problems. Their job was to work together and choose the supplements that would be safe and effective for their theoretical patients. The level of confusion and frustration that accompanied their collective foraging through rows and rows of products was high, to say the least. These health-care professionals with more than one year of advanced training in integrative medicine struggled mightily to make sense of all the different dietary supplement products. So, if you've ever found yourself standing in the supplement aisle of a store, looking at all the bottles on the shelf, feeling absolutely bewildered by the endless array of choices, you are definitely not alone.

You're an intelligent person. You should be able to turn that supplement bottle around, read the label and understand what it's saying. Right? Don't bet on it. The dietary supplement industry has not made it easy to figure out what you are buying. Consider vitamin B12: It is available as a single supplement in doses ranging from 25 mcg to 1,000 mcg. That's a very big range! Taking 25 to 50 mcg is sufficient for most people, but if you're deficient in B12, taking 500 to 1,000 mcg per day would make sense. B12 is also sold in combination with other B-vitamins as part of a B-complex supplement—or as part of a multivitamin-mineral supplement. Taking the B-vitamins together enhances their effectiveness, so either of these products would be a good choice, especially if you are taking a high dose of vitamin B12 by itself to correct a low level. B12 is often featured in products that contain various vitamins, minerals, amino acids, and herbs designed to help improve your memory or energy. Look carefully at all the other ingredients. Are they really necessary? Would any of them interact with your medications? Also, vitamin B12 is commonly found in supplements in the form of cyanocobalamin or methylcobalamin. Is one form better than the other? Although many people are able to convert cyanocobalamin to methylcobalamin, the active form of B12 in the body, what if you're one of those who can't (which you would only know through sophisticated lab testing)? Taking methylcobalamin is the better option. As you can see, even with something as simple as vitamin B12, there is a lot to think about, isn't there?

As for minerals, maybe you've read that magnesium is good for preventing migraine headaches. And indeed it is! You go to the store and look at the magnesium section. Do you take magnesium alone or with calcium? Is there a difference between magnesium oxide, citrate, lactate, malate, and glycinate? Is one better than another? Will magnesium supplementation interfere with any of your prescription medications? When should you take this supplement, and in what dosage? Whew!

Then there is what I call fluff in many supplements. These are ingredients that sound impressive on the label but in actuality the product contains so little of them that they have no beneficial effect on your health. While you might feel warm and fuzzy when the label says, "Contains real blueberries!" you probably wouldn't feel that way if you knew that the 50 mg of freeze-dried powder it contains is equivalent to roughly one blueberry. That's right. It takes *22,000 mg* of freeze-dried blueberry powder to equal 1 cup of fresh blueberries. I'm not sure that one solitary blueberry is going to do you that much good. It's marketing fluff.

My family rolls their eyes when we're strolling through our local natural foods grocery and I notice someone looking puzzled in the supplement aisle. Try as I might to just keep shopping, I feel an overwhelming urge to go help the person. I know all too well how frustrating it can be for most people to read a supplement label and try to decipher what it means.

Besides figuring out what supplements you need, you also want to try to determine the quality of those supplements. Most of the really disturbing news about "supplements" is not about vitamins, minerals, or common nutritional supplements, which generally contain what they claim on their labels. The really problematic supplements are typically those associated with weight loss, body-building, and sexual enhancement. Steer clear of these categories. Herbal products coming out of China and India have been found on numerous occasions to be adulterated with undeclared prescription drugs, as well as containing high levels of lead, mercury, and/or arsenic. Stick with large reputable brands sold by natural foods groceries and manufactured in the U.S.

There are also broader questions to consider when it comes to nutritional supplements. When you look closely at the label, you might find ingredients that you would never consume if they were listed on a food label. You want to make sure the supplements you take are consistent with your values when it comes to organic, non-GMO ingredients, allergens, and/or artificial preservatives and colorings.

I understand the issues you're wrestling with, because I've been working in this field for more than 30 years. I want to help demystify the supplement aisle so that you can feel more confident when you are shopping for you and your family.

First, let me help you get some clarity about what types of nutritional supplements are out there: vitamins, minerals, botanicals, and everything else.

VITAMINS AND MINERALS

The word *vitamin,* originally spelled *vitamine,* comes from the root words *vita,* meaning "life," and *amine,* which refers to organic compounds that are derivatives of ammonia (for example, amino acids). Once we learned that not all vitamins are amines, the *e* was dropped. However, one thing remains true: Vitamins are absolutely essential for life. They are necessary for producing energy, preventing damage to our DNA, regulating cell and tissue growth, and much more.

There are 13 essential vitamins: A, C, D, E, K, B1 (thiamine), B2 (riboflavin), B3 (niacin), B5 (pantothenic acid), B6 (pyridoxine), B7 (biotin), B9 (folate, or folic acid), and B12 (cobalamin). Vitamins are further divided into fat-soluble (A, D, E, K) and water-soluble (the other nine). Your body can technically make vitamins D and K; the rest absolutely must be obtained in the diet. This is why it is so important to eat a varied diet that can provide what your body needs on a regular basis.

Minerals are elements that originate in the earth. Plants absorb minerals from the soil, and when animals or humans eat the plants, they ingest the minerals, as well. The mineral content in food varies considerably based upon geographical location and soil quality. The major minerals necessary for health are calcium, magnesium, phosphorous, sodium, potassium, chloride, and sulfur. You also need trace minerals, so named because they are needed only in very small amounts. The primary trace minerals include iron, zinc, iodine, selenium, copper, manganese, fluoride, chromium, and molybdenum. The body cannot make any of these minerals; they must be obtained through food.

In nature, minerals are generally bound to another substance. Calcium bound to carbonate is found in limestone, chalk, coral and many other natural substances. Calcium in dietary supplements is also bound to other substances, which can occur naturally or be produced in the laboratory. The substance a mineral is bound to can impact its absorption and bioavailability. Calcium carbonate is widely used in supplements but is poorly absorbed in those with little stomach acid. Calcium hydroxyapatite is made from bovine bone. The hydroxyapatite fraction contains phosphorous, zinc, magnesium and other minerals typically found in bone. Some people object to supplementing with ground bone. Calcium citrate and calcium malate are produced in the laboratory and are generally well absorbed in supplements. We'll discuss the optimal forms for taking minerals in Chapter 5.

A wholesome diet rich in vegetables, fruits, nuts, seeds, beans, dairy, eggs, seafood, and grass-fed meat, along with some iodized salt, can provide all the nutrients you need, with the possible exception of vitamin D. But having cared for many people over the years, I can honestly say that this just isn't the way most Americans eat. That is why I believe many people would benefit from taking a basic multivitamin-mineral supplement, particularly women who could become or are pregnant or nursing; children under the age of five (especially if they are picky eaters . . . or picky eaters of any age, for that matter), vegetarians/vegans, those over the age of fifty, and people who have certain medical conditions or are taking prescription medications.

OTHER NUTRITIONAL SUPPLEMENTS

There are many nutritional supplements in the marketplace besides vitamins and minerals. Some substances are "essential," meaning your body absolutely requires that you get them in your diet, or in a supplement, because your body cannot produce them. Examples include omega-3 fatty acids and the nine essential amino acids, such as lysine and tryptophan. Substances that are not essential in the diet but are highly beneficial include phytonutrients (nutrients from plants); probiotics (microorganisms that help with digestion); prebiotics (dietary fiber that promotes development of a healthy population of microorganism in the digestive system); and dozens of others. There are also substances that are produced in the human body that can be taken in supplement form such as melatonin, coenzyme Q10, glucosamine, and chondroitin. These various supplements are often lumped into an umbrella category referred to as nutraceuticals. There is no legal or regulatory definition for what constitutes a nutraceutical, but the term is loosely used in the supplement industry to describe all the dietary supplements that are not vitamins, minerals, or herbal supplements. Some nutraceuticals can play an important role in maintaining your health or treating a specific health condition. In Chapter 6, you'll learn about some of the more common nutraceuticals that I recommend to my patients.

The last category of dietary supplements is botanical or herbal medicines. I admit that I am passionate about this topic, which is why I wrote about them at length in my book *Healthy at Home* and in the *National Geographic Guide to Medicinal Herbs,* which I co-authored. There are many ways to experience the benefits of herbs in your life. Culinary herbs and spices are an inexpensive and healthy way to greatly enhance the flavor of food without increasing salt intake or calories. And they are also powerhouse medicines! Garlic, onions, cinnamon, turmeric, ginger, basil, thyme, and oregano can all dial back inflammation, counter oxidative stress, maintain blood sugar levels, aid digestion, rev up the immune system, and much more. Gentle remedies, such as chamomile, lemon balm, peppermint, and passionflower, can soothe the nerves, ease anxiety, promote restful sleep, and settle an upset tummy. I firmly believe that many of the plants that have been used as food and medicine for thousands of years can be an effective strategy for fortifying your life today. But herbal medicine is a huge topic and since I've already written about it in my previous books, in this book, I am going to focus my attention on the foundational supplements, principally vitamins, minerals, and some key nutraceuticals.

Now it's time to look at a typical supplement label so that I can explain all the pieces. We'll also explore some key issues you'll want to consider regarding quality, dose, safe upper limits, dissolution, and bioavailability.

ANATOMY OF A DIETARY SUPPLEMENT LABEL

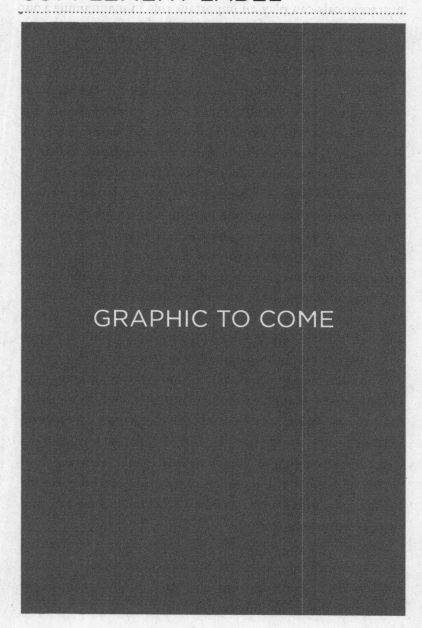

1. PRODUCT NAME

The product name can be anything from a single ingredient (vitamin D), to a combination of ingredients (calcium with vitamin D), to a catchy name that hints at what the product does (bone strength). Always make sure you read the ingredient section carefully. For instance, when you purchase a product with the words vitamin D in large print on the front of the label, you want to know if it contains cholecalciferol (D3) or ergocalciferol (D2), the latter being less potent than the former. Both, however, are technically vitamin D.

Manufacturers often design products for a specific health issue or for a certain group of people, such as women, or adults over the age of 50. Here again, read the label carefully and remember one size doesn't fit all. Let's say you're a 35-year-old woman standing in the supplement aisle looking at dozens of women's multivitamin-mineral products. You see that there is a Women's Multi and a Women's Multi 55 Plus. You choose the Women's Multi because of your age. This supplement provides 100 percent of the daily value (more on that later) for iron. But let's assume you had a hysterectomy last year and are no longer having menstrual periods. A woman who is not menstruating, pregnant or breastfeeding should not take supplemental iron unless instructed to by a health-care professional. The Women's Multi 55 Plus doesn't contain iron, as it assumes a 55-year-old woman would no longer be having periods. In this case, the 55 Plus product would be a better choice. Read the labels carefully and do your homework (which you're doing by reading this book!), so that you know what you need and know exactly what you are buying.

2. MANUFACTURER'S NAME

Manufacturers are required to provide their name. This is in part to ensure that if there is an adverse event, such as vomiting or a severe rash after taking the supplement, you and your health-care provider know who to contact for more information or to report the incident. Manufacturers are required by law to report any serious adverse events to the FDA within 15 days. If you have questions about a product, don't hesitate to contact the company. See "12. Manufacturer's Contact Information" on page XX for more about how to get in touch with a manufacturer.

3. MANUFACTURER'S CLAIMS

The Food and Drug Administration (FDA) has strict rules about what companies can say about supplements. Manufacturers can claim that a supplement supports general well-being or the normal structure or function of the human body. For instance, such statements as "Calcium builds strong bones" or "Antioxidants maintain cell integrity" are permitted. However, labels (and advertisements) cannot claim that the supplement treats or cures diseases. So, while there are randomized controlled trials demonstrating that the herb St. John's wort is effective for the treatment of mild forms of depression, a manufacturer cannot say this on the label. Instead, the label would have to say something like "St. John's wort supports a healthy mood." The regulatory system for claims is far from ideal, but it would be chaos if manufacturers could make disease claims not substantiated by science.

While not technically a "claim," *many* companies make sure their labels include mention of minuscule amounts of herbs and/or foods included in their supplements. These ingredients are neither harmful nor helpful but are given catchy phrases that sound good for marketing purposes. Remember what I said about 50 mg of "freeze-dried blueberry" being less than one actual blueberry? Another example is a supplement that contains 125 mg of a "food blend" of spinach, dandelion leaves, burdock root, and carrots. Now, that might look good on the label, but to have any beneficial effect, you would need *grams* of *each* of these ingredients. Don't pay a premium price for marketing extras like these.

4. METHOD OF DELIVERY

Dietary supplements (DS) can come in a variety of forms, such as tablets, capsules, softgels, chewables, lozenges, powders, or liquids. There are advantages and disadvantages for each.

Tablets: Generally, tablets are a cost-effective way to take supplements, as ingredients can be tightly packed, allowing for higher potency options. Tablets are shelf-stable and have longer expiration dates. If you have a healthy digestive tract and are not taking such medications as proton pump inhibitors (Nexium, Prilosec) that shut off your production of stomach acid, your digestive system shouldn't have any problem breaking down a supplement tablet made by a reputable manufacturer. Those taking proton pump inhibitors might want to consider taking capsules, softgels, liquids, or powders.

The primary downside is that large tablets can be difficult to swallow. Pill-swallowing cups are designed to help you swallow medications and supplements and can be purchased at most drugstores. You can also use a pill slicer to cut your tablets in half, which makes them smaller but also leaves a rough edge that can irritate your throat.

Note: It's important that you don't grind or split a tablet that is enteric-coated, such as SAMe (used for arthritis and depression) or peppermint oil (used for irritable bowel syndrome). The coating is designed to prevent/slow its dissolution in the stomach to ensure optimal benefit of the ingredients.

If you do purchase a supplement with tablets that are just too large to swallow, take it back and exchange it for one that you can actually take. Ask the store clerk or pharmacist to help you find a similar product made as "mini-tabs," capsules, chewables, or liquid.

Tablets require binders and fillers to hold them together and make them a uniform size. Manufacturers sometimes use dyes to make the tablets look more appealing. Some people may object to, or be allergic to, some of these binders, fillers, or colorings. A more complete discussion on this topic is found under "9: Other Ingredients," on page XX.

Capsules: Most of us are familiar with two-piece gelatin capsules that are widely used for supplements and prescription drugs. Many supplement manufacturers use capsules made from vegetable material (veggie caps) but some may contain gelatin derived from animals—something vegetarians/vegans will want to watch for on the label. Capsules are easy to swallow and break down quickly in the stomach. You can also open the capsule and put the ingredients into a smoothie, applesauce, or yogurt, making capsules an attractive option for children or those who have difficulty swallowing. Capsules do not need binders, as tablets do, but they do often contain nonactive substances that prevent the ingredients from clumping and caking. They also often need fillers to top up the capsule: to make it completely full. Most capsules are designed to hold 400 to 500 mg of powdered ingredients. A manufacturer creating capsules that deliver 125 mg of a nutrient or herb has to add 375 mg of filler. This is often rice powder, which is hypoallergenic and well tolerated by most. When you're buying supplements in capsules, read the "other ingredients" section carefully so you know what fillers, if any, were used. Also keep in mind that capsules have a shorter shelf life than tablets because they are not airtight. In general, they are more expensive and less potent than tablets because the ingredients cannot be so tightly compressed.

Softgels: These are smooth, soft, one-piece capsules designed to hold liquid or oil-based preparations, such as vitamin E or fish oil. Unlike capsules, they are currently made almost exclusively from gelatin from animal sources, so vegetarians/vegans take note. Softgels are easy to swallow and, because they are airtight, offer a long shelf life. The primary downside is the cost, as they are more expensive to produce.

Chewables: If you like to take your supplements in the form of gummy bears, don't be embarrassed. You aren't the only one! Chewables are one of the fastest growing categories of dietary supplements. They generally command a higher price and most contain some form of sugar, sweetener, and/or flavoring, which could be natural or artificial—so read the label closely. Many higher quality supplements are using such sweeteners as stevia, xylitol, or erythritol that do not impact blood sugar or cause tooth decay. Prolonged use of high-potency chewable vitamin C (500 mg), however, has been associated with erosion of tooth enamel, so I don't recommend them except for occasional use. Make sure you keep chewable supplements away from youngsters who may confuse them with candy. Vegans and those sensitive to dairy should take note that some chewable supplements contain lactic acid, which may have been derived from dairy.

Lozenges: Small tablets designed to dissolve slowly in the mouth, lozenges are generally used to soothe a cough or sore throat. Some vitamin or mineral supplements are available in lozenge form, as an alternative to chewables. Many lozenges contain some type of sweetener and may also contain flavorings and colorings, so read the label carefully. Lozenges are generally reasonably priced. Keep them away from young children that may confuse them with candy.

Powders: Powders are useful when you want to use larger amounts of a supplement. For example, the amount of inositol generally used for anxiety or sleep is typically 6 to 12 grams, or 2 to 4 teaspoons. That would be anywhere from 12 to 24 capsules per day! Powdered supplements are good for those who don't like to take or have difficulty swallowing pills, as they are easily added to smoothies and food. Supplement powders are generally best when mixed with cool, room-temperature, or warm liquids (below 120°F). Prolonged exposure to high temperatures will destroy water-soluble vitamins, but fat-soluble vitamins and minerals are generally fine. Powders offer a pretty good value and have a decent shelf life as long as you store them in an airtight container in a cool, dark place. The downside is that you have to put them into something you will consume, making them less convenient when traveling or on the go.

Liquids: Liquid supplements are another option for those who prefer not to take pills or capsules. Some vitamins and minerals are available in a sublingual form, drops (or sometimes small quickly dissolving tabs) that are placed under the tongue for rapid absorption. A classic example is vitamin B12. The base for a liquid supplement varies considerably ranging from water and vegetable glycerin to coconut water or juice. Many contain sweeteners and flavorings. Some products, such as fish or cod liver oil, may contain only the ingredient and some natural flavoring. Liquids allow a great deal of flexibility when it comes to dosing, and you don't have to worry about absorption issues. They can be ideal for children and those who have difficulty swallowing. The downsides are that they are more expensive, have a shorter shelf life, are harder to transport—and many need to be refrigerated after opening. Always shake liquid supplements before use, as some ingredients may settle on the bottom of the bottle.

Topicals: Many creams, gels, lotions, ointments, and liniments contain vitamins, minerals, nutraceuticals, and herbal ingredients. Many people open a vitamin E capsule and apply it to prevent scarring when skin has been injured. Epsom salts can deliver magnesium through the skin and relax sore muscles. Calendula ointment is commonly used for minor cuts and wounds. However, topically applied products are not technically considered dietary supplements and are not regulated as such.

WARNING!
IV Nutrition

Intravenous drips (IVs) of specific vitamins or minerals are used both inside and outside of a hospital setting to provide nutrition directly into the bloodstream. IV-administered nutrients are not considered dietary supplements and should only be used under the supervision of an appropriately trained health-care professional.

---

5. "SUPPLEMENT FACTS" OR INGREDIENTS

The supplement facts panel includes a list of all the ingredients in the product. You will see the list of ingredients under "Amount Per Serving." It should provide specific information about the particular nutrient, such as vitamin D (as cholecalciferol) or vitamin B12 (as methylcobalamin). If the label doesn't show this detailed specification right next to the nutrient, you will need to look further down the label and try to sort out what form of nutrient is being used in the product. This makes it much more difficult for consumers to know *exactly* what they are getting. If you can't find the specific form of the ingredient that is used in the supplement, check the manufacturer's website or better yet, just purchase a higher-quality supplement!

6. SERVING INFORMATION

While it might seem odd to refer to a capsule or tablet as a serving size, supplements are regulated like food, not drugs. This section of the label tells you how many capsules/tablets or how much liquid or powder you will need to take to reach the amount listed on the label. Read this carefully and compare your options. Do you really want to take six tablets everyday, when you can get the same essential ingredient in another formulation that requires you take only two? Additionally, this section of the label will tell you how many servings the manufacturer recommends you take each day. It may also suggest when to take the supplement, for instance, "Take one tablet twice daily with meals."

Figuring out how much of a certain supplement *you* should take is important, regardless of the manufacturer's recommendations. When it comes to vitamins and minerals, we have a pretty good idea about how much is needed to prevent frank disease. Most of us, however, would like to do more than just prevent rickets or beriberi; we would like to experience vitality and health. But just as important, you'll want to make sure that you are not taking *too much* of any particular ingredient or nutrient. You must take into account your age, gender, diet, and a host of other factors. I'll give you some specifics about amounts under "8: Percentage of Daily Value," on page XX.

7. UNITS OF MEASUREMENT

In general, in the United States, international unit (IU) is the typical standard unit of measure for fat-soluble vitamins (A, D, and E). Milligram (mg) and microgram (mcg) are standard units of measure for the other vitamins and minerals. One microgram is equal to .001 milligrams. One milligram is equal to .001 grams.

8. PERCENTAGE/DAILY VALUE

The daily value (DV) is a percentage, calculated on the *average* recommended daily allowance (RDA) for adults. For each nutrient, there is only one DV for everyone four years of age and older. That means the DV does not distinguish between the nutritional needs of an 80-year-old man, a 29-year-old woman, or a 6-year-old child. Be aware that your RDA might be higher or lower than the DV. For example, the DV for vitamin D is 400 IU, whereas the RDA for anyone from 12 months to 70 years of age is 600 IU—and 800 IU if you're over the age of 70. All vitamins will list 400 IU as 100 percent of the DV, yet just as an example of how general the DV is, a 75-year-old man would actually need double that amount. Ingredients that do not have a daily value will have an asterisk (*) in the DV column and generally fall into the herbal and nutraceutical categories.

So, those are the basics for understanding what is on the supplement label. Now I would like to talk a bit more about some other terms that are important for you to understand and how they apply to you.

The RDA is the amount of a vitamin or mineral that the Food and Nutrition Board, which is part of the Institute of Medicine at the National Academy of Science, considers sufficient for ingestion in one day. The first RDAs were established in 1941 and they are reviewed and revised every 5 to 10 years. The adequate intake (AI) is used when there is not enough information to determine an RDA. This level is expected to meet the needs necessary for "maintaining health." What *you* need to maintain health may differ depending on your individual health goals and unique needs.

The DV, as described previously, is what you will see on dietary supplement labels. The DV is based upon the RDAs that were set in 1968. That is why the DV for vitamin D is still 400 IU, even though the RDA was increased to 600 to 800 IU in 2010. It's confusing, I know. Again, for each nutrient, there is only *one* DV for everyone four years of age and older. Keep this in mind when reading your supplement label!

Important note: What you will *not* see on the label is information about the upper limit (UL), which is the tolerable upper intake level for a given nutrient. In other words, the UL is the

Daily Values

Vitamin A	5,000 International Unites (IU)
Vitamin C	60 mg
Calcium	1,000 mg
Iron	18 mg
Vitamin D	400 IU
Vitamin E	30 IU
Vitamin K	80 micrograms μg
Thiamin	1.5 mg
Riboflavin	1.7 mg
Niacin	20 mg
Vitamin B6	2 mg
Folate	400 μg
Vitamin B12	6 μg
Biotin	300 μg
Pantothentic acid	10 mg
Phosphorus	1,000 mg
Iodine	150 μg
Magnesium	400 mg
Zinc	15 mg
Selenium	70 μg
Copper	2 mg
Manganese	2mg
Chromium	120 μg
Molybdenum	75 μg
Chloride	3,400 mg

highest daily intake of a particular nutrient unlikely to pose a risk of adverse health effects to almost all people in the general population, as determined by the Food and Nutrition Board. Please hear me when I say that more is *not* always better. I have *never* been a fan of "mega-dose" supplements. It's too easy to take more than you need, which can lead to problems. The UL represents the *total* intake from food, beverages, and supplements, with one important exception: magnesium. The UL only applies to magnesium in dietary supplements. On the charts that follow, it's important to note that just because a vitamin or mineral has the designation ND (meaning the upper limit is *not determinable*) instead of a UL, it doesn't mean that it is safe to take in infinite amounts. ND just means we lack data regarding adverse health effects in a particular age group for a particular nutrient. (I will go into more detail about safe ranges of individual vitamins and minerals in Chapters 4 and 5.)

WARNING!
Beware of Supplement Overload

The very young and the very old, along with people who have diminished kidney and liver capacity due to disease or aging, must be extra careful with supplements. The kidneys and liver are vital organs for eliminating what the body doesn't need. Overloading them with too much of anything makes it harder for them to do their job. Medications and supplements can build up in your system, causing problems. If you're pregnant, breastfeeding, elderly, or choosing supplements for a young child, be especially careful about staying within daily intake ranges for given nutrients. When in doubt, talk to a qualified health-care practitioner!

Tolerable Upper Intake for Vitamins and Minerals

Dietary Reference Intakes (DRIs): Tolerable Upper Intake Levels, Vitamins
Food and Nutrition Board, Institute of Medicine, National Academies

Life Stage Group	Vitamin A (µ g/d)[1]	Vitamin C (mg/d)	Vitamin D (µ g/d)	Vitamin E (mg/d)[2, 3]	Vitamin K	Thiamin	Ribo-flavin
Infants							
0 to 6 mo	600	ND[5]	25	ND	ND	ND	ND
6 to 12 mo	600	ND	38	ND	ND	ND	ND
Children							
1-3 y	600	400	63	200	ND	ND	ND
4-8 y	900	650	75	300	ND	ND	ND
Males							
9-13 y	1,700	1,200	100	600	ND	ND	ND
14-18 y	2,800	1,800	100	800	ND	ND	ND
19-30 y	3,000	2,000	100	1,000	ND	ND	ND
31-50 y	3,000	2,000	100	1,000	ND	ND	ND
51-70 y	3,000	2,000	100	1,000	ND	ND	ND
>70 y	3,000	2,000	100	1,000	ND	ND	ND
Females							
9-13 y	1,700	1,200	100	600	ND	ND	ND
14-18 y	2,800	1,800	100	800	ND	ND	ND
19-30 y	3,000	2,000	100	1,000	ND	ND	ND
31-50 y	3,000	2,000	100	1,000	ND	ND	ND
51-70 y	3,000	2,000	100	1,000	ND	ND	ND
>70 y	3,000	2,000	100	1,000	ND	ND	ND
Pregnancy							
14-18 y	2,800	1,800	100	800	ND	ND	ND
19-30 y	3,000	2,000	100	1,000	ND	ND	ND
31-50 y	3,000	2,000	100	1,000	ND	ND	ND
Lactation							
14-18 y	2,800	1,800	100	800	ND	ND	ND
19-30 y	3,000	2,000	100	1,000	ND	ND	ND
31-50 y	3,000	2,000	100	1,000	ND	ND	ND

NOTE: A Tolerable Upper Intake Level (UL) is the highest level of daily nutrient intake that is likely to pose no risk of adverse health effects to almost all individuals in the general population. Unless otherwise specified, the UL represents total intake from food, water, and supplements. Due to lack of suitable data, ULs could not be established for vitamin K, thiamin, riboflavin, vitamin B[12], pantothenic acid, biotin, and carotenoids. In the absence of a UL, extra caution may be warranted in consuming levels above recommended intakes. Members of the general population should be advised not to routinely exceed the UL. The UL is not meant to apply to individuals who are treated with the nutrient under medical supervision or to individuals with predisposing conditions that modify their sensitivity to the nutrient.

Niacin (mg/d)[c]	Vitamin B$_6$ (mg/d)	Folate (μg/d)[c]	Vitamin B$_{12}$	Panto-thenic Acid	Bio-tin	Cho-line (g/d)	Carote-noids[4]
ND	ND	ND	ND	ND	ND	ND	ND
ND	ND	ND	ND	ND	ND	ND	ND
10	30	300	ND	ND	ND	1.0	ND
15	40	400	ND	ND	ND	1.0	ND
20	60	600	ND	ND	ND	2.0	ND
30	80	800	ND	ND	ND	3.0	ND
35	100	1,000	ND	ND	ND	3.5	ND
35	.100	1,000	ND	ND	ND	3.5	ND
35	100	1,000	ND	ND	ND	3.5	ND
35	100	1,000	ND	ND	ND	3.5	ND
20	60	600	ND	ND	ND	2.0	ND
30	80	800	ND	ND	ND	3.0	ND
35	100	1,000	ND	ND	ND	3.5	ND
35	100	1,000	ND	ND	ND	3.5	ND
35	100	1,000	ND	ND	ND	3.5	ND
35	100	1,000	ND	ND	ND	3.5	ND
30	80	800	ND	ND	ND	3.0	ND
35	100	1,000	ND	ND	ND	3.5	ND
35	100	1,000	ND	ND	ND	3.5	ND
30	80	800	ND	ND	ND	3.0	ND
35	100	1,000	ND	ND	ND	3.5	ND
35	100	1,000	ND	ND	ND	3.5	ND

SOURCES: *Dietary Reference Intakes for Calcium, Phosphorus, Magnesium, Vitamin D, and Fluoride* (1997); *Dietary Reference Intakes for Thiamin, Riboflavin, Niacin, Vitamin B$_6$, Folate, Vitamin B$_{12}$, Pantothenic Acid, Biotin, and Choline* (1998); *Dietary Reference Intakes for Vitamin C, Vitamin E, Selenium, and Carotenoids* (2000); *Dietary Reference Intakes for Vitamin A, Vitamin K, Arsenic, Boron, Chromium, Copper, Iodine, Iron, Manganese, Molybdenum, Nickel, Silicon, Vanadium, and Zinc* (2001); and *Dietary Reference Intakes for Calcium and Vitamin D* (2011). These reports may be accessed via www.nap.edu.

Dietary Reference Intakes (DRIs): Tolerable Upper Intake Levels, Elements

Food and Nutrition Board, Institute of Medicine, National Academies

Life Stage Group	Arsenic[6]	Boron (mg/d)	Calcium (mg/d)	Chro-mium	Copper (µg/d)	Flouride (mg/d)	Iodine (µg/d)	Iron (mg/d)	Magnesium[7] (mg/d)	
Infants										
0 to 6 mo	ND[10]	ND	1,000	ND	ND	0.7	ND	40	ND	
6 to 12 mo	ND	ND	1,500	ND	ND	0.9	ND	40	ND	
Children										
1-3 y	ND	3	2,500	ND	1,000	1.3	200	40	65	
4-8 y	ND	6	2,500	ND	3,000	2.2	300	40	110	
Males										
9-13 y	ND	11	3,000	ND	5,000	10	600	40	350	
14-18 y	ND	17	3,000	ND	8,000	10	900	45	350	
19-30 y	ND	20	2,500	ND	10,000	10	1,100	45	350	
31-50 y	ND	20	2,500	ND	10,000	10	1,100	45	350	
51-70 y	ND	20	2,000	ND	10,000	10	1,100	45	350	
>70 y	ND	20	2,000	ND	10,000	10	1,100	45	350	
Females										
9-13 y	ND	11	3,000	ND	5,000	10	600	40	350	
14-18 y	ND	17	3,000	ND	8,000	10	900	45	350	
19-30 y	ND	20	2,500	ND	10,000	10	1,100	45	350	
31-50 y	ND	20	2,500	ND	10,000	10	1,100	45	350	
51-70 y	ND	20	2,000	ND	10,000	10	1,100	45	350	
>70 y	ND	20	2,000	ND	10,000	10	1,100	45	350	
Pregnancy										
14-18 y	ND	17	3,000	ND	8,000	10	900	45	350	
19-30 y	ND	20	2,500	ND	10,000	10	1,100	45	350	
31-50 y	ND	20	2,500	ND	10,000	10	1,100	45	350	
Lactation										
14-18 y	ND	17	3,000	ND	8,000	10	900	45	350	
19-30 y	ND	20	2,500	ND	10,000	10	1,100	45	350	
31-50 y	ND	20	2,500	ND	10,000	10	1,100	45	350	

NOTE: A Tolerable Upper Intake Level (UL) is the highest level of daily nutrient intake that is likely to pose no risk of adverse health effects to almost all individuals in the general population. Unless otherwise specified, the UL represents total intake from food, water, and supplements. Due to lack of suitable data, ULs could not be established for vitamin K, thiamin, riboflavin, vitamin B_{12}, pantothenic acid, biotin, and carotenoids. In the absence of a UL, extra caution may be warranted in consuming levels above recommended intakes. Members of the general population should be advised not to routinely exceed the UL. The UL is not meant to apply to individuals who are treated with the nutrient under medical supervision or to individuals with predisposing conditions that modify their sensitivity to the nutrient.

SOURCES: *Dietary Reference Intakes for Calcium, Phosphorus, Magnesium, Vitamin D, and Fluoride* (1997); *Dietary Reference Intakes for Thiamin, Riboflavin, Niacin, Vitamin B_6, Folate, Vitamin B_{12}, Pantothenic Acid, Biotin, and Choline* (1998); *Dietary Reference Intakes for Vitamin C, Vitamin E, Selenium, and Carotenoids* (2000); *Dietary Reference Intakes for Vitamin A, Vitamin K, Arsenic, Boron, Chromium, Copper, Iodine, Iron, Manganese, Molybdenum, Nickel, Silicon, Vanadium, and Zinc* (2001); and *Dietary Reference Intakes for Calcium and Vitamin D* (2011). These reports may be accessed via www.nap.edu.

Manganese (mg/d)	Molybdenum (µ g/s)	Nickel (mg/d)	Phosphorus (g/d)	Selenium	Silicon[8]	Vanadium[9] (mg/d)	Zinc (mg/d)	Sodium (g/d)	Chloride (g/d)
ND	ND	ND	ND	45	ND	ND	4	ND	ND
ND	ND	ND	ND	60	ND	ND	5	ND	ND
2	300	0.2	3	90	ND	ND	7	1.5	2.3
3	600	0.3	3	150	ND	ND	12	1.9	2.9
6	1,100	0.6	4	280	ND	ND	23	2.2	3.4
9	1,700	1.0	4	400	ND	ND	34	2.3	3.6
11	2,000	1.0	4	400	ND	1.8	40	2.3	3.6
11	2,000	1.0	4	400	ND	1.8	40	2.3	3.6
11	2,000	1.0	4	400	ND	1.8	40	2.3	3.6
11	2,000	1.0	3	400	ND	1.8	40	2.3	3.6
6	1,100	0.6	4	280	ND	ND	23	2.2	3.4
9	1,700	1.0	4	400	ND	ND	34	2.3	3.6
11	2,000	1.0	4	400	ND	1.8	40	2.3	3.6
11	2,000	1.0	4	400	ND	1.8	40	2.3	3.6
11	2,000	1.0	4	400	ND	1.8	40	2.3	3.6
11	2,000	1.0	3	400	ND	1.8	40	2.3	3.6
9	1,700	1.0	3.5	400	ND	ND	34	2.3	3.6
11	2,000	1.0	3.5	400	ND	ND	40	2.3	3.6
11	2,000	1.0	3.5	400	ND	ND	40	2.3	3.6
9	1,700	1.0	4	400	ND	ND	34	2.3	3.6
11	2,000	1.0	4	400	ND	ND	40	2.3	3.6
11	2,000	1.0	4	400	ND	ND	40	2.3	3.6

1   As performed vitamin A only.

2   As α-tocopherol; applies to any form of supplemental α-tocopherol.

3   The ULs for vitamin E, niacin, and folate apply to synthetic forms obtained from supplements, fortified foods, or a combination of the two.

4   B-Carotene supplements are advised only to serve as a provitamin A source for individuals at risk of vitamin deficiency.

5   ND = Not determinable due to lack of data of adverse effects in this age group and concern with regard to lack of ability to handle excess amounts. Source of intake should be from food only to prevent high levels of intake.

6   Although the UL was not determined for arsenic, there is no justification for adding arsenic to food or supplements.

7   The ULs for magnesium represent intake from a pharmacological agent only and do not include intake from food and water.

8   Although silicon has not been shown to cause adverse effect in humans, there is no justification for adding silicon to supplements.

9   Although vanadium in food has not been shown to cause adverse effects in humans, there is no justification for adding vanadium to food and vanadium supplements should be used with caution. The UL is based on adverse effects in laboratory animals and this data could be used to set a UL for adults but not children and adolescents.

10   ND = Not determinable due to lack of data of adverse effects in this age group and concern with regard to lack of ability to handle excess amounts. Source of intake should be from food only to prevent high levels of intake.

9. OTHER INGREDIENTS

The "other ingredients" section is where you will find the nonactive ingredients (excipients) listed, including any binders, fillers, colorings, or solvents. These ingredients are often included to ensure tablet integrity, proper dissolution, or shelf life. It is particularly important to review this part of the label if you have an allergy (for example, to soy or gluten), but also because some of these ingredients may not be consistent with your values when it comes to artificial ingredients, non-GMO products, et cetera, which are often used in cheaper mass-produced brands. Rarely can you determine whether certain ingredients are from genetically modified sources, without doing research beyond reading the label. While the FDA has worked to make label information clearer whether components in food or supplements might be associated with allergies, there are still problems. Following are some of the most commonly used excipients in the industry.

Flow Agents

Flow agents are used to help in the manufacturing of tablets and capsules, to prevent ingredients from clumping and caking. Vegetarian sources commonly include silicon dioxide, magnesium stearate, and stearic acid. I will discuss each of them briefly. Silicon occurs naturally in foods as silicon dioxide, silica, and silicates. After reviewing the evidence, the European Food Safety Authority concluded that up to 1,500 mg per day of silicon dioxide added to food supplements is of no safety concern. Manufacturers use far less.

Magnesium stearate, a combination of magnesium and stearic acid, is one of the most commonly used excipients and one of the most vilified. Magnesium is an essential mineral, important for your health. Stearic acid is found in many common foods, such as flaxseed oil, walnut oil, olive oil, beef, lamb, and chocolate. Humans regularly consume it in relatively high amounts: A chocolate bar contains roughly 5,000 mg. A supplement typically contains only 20 to 50 mg, so why all the hoopla? Two small studies suggested that when large doses of stearic acid were added to petri dishes containing immune cells taken from mice, it damaged them. This doesn't really mean much—drip enough of almost anything onto cells in petri dish and you'll damage them. The small amounts of magnesium stearate in a supplement will not harm you or your immune system. That said, some studies suggest that it can slow the disintegration of tablets, which might be a problem if your digestive system isn't working optimally or if you are taking medications that shut down stomach acid. The bigger issue is the source of stearic acid, which is often derived from palm oil harvested from tropical rainforests. Some environmental groups are asking people to cut back on the use of palm oil due to loss of rain forest habitat. You need to be aware of the issues so that you can make choices based upon both the science and your values.

Binders

Binders allow the ingredients in a tablet to stick together and not crumble. Most are vegetarian friendly and none are considered problematic. One of the more common binders is cellulose, or microcrystalline cellulose, which is derived from wood pulp. Guar gum, xanthan gum, and acacia gum, also very common, are all derived from plants.

Fillers

When the ingredient amount is very small—for example, in microgram quantities (iodine, folic acid, selenium, and so on)—fillers are used to top off the capsule. Rice flour is most typically used because it is hypoallergenic, but cornstarch, lactose, or other potential allergens could be present. Read the label carefully.

Coating Agents

Coating agents are used to coat tablets, helping to bind the ingredients and make tablets smooth and easier to swallow. Lecithin, made from soy, is often used as a coating agent. Studies show that soy lecithin products can vary considerably in the amount of protein they contain. If you have a serious soy allergy and are concerned, avoid products that list lecithin on the label. Sometimes the label will list vegetable glaze or vegetable coating, which could be derived from corn—a problem for some people and also possibly genetically modified. Modified cellulose, derived from wood pulp, is also used to coat tablets and may be listed as hydroxypropyl methylcellulose (HPMC).

Acidulants

To prevent microbes from growing in liquid products and spoiling them, acidulants, such as citric acid, malic acid, tartaric acid, and aspartic acid, are often used. The only one that might be problematic is aspartic acid, a nonessential amino acid also found in aspartame. While the amount of aspartic acid present in a dietary supplement is very small, some people can be quite sensitive and might experience headaches or stomach discomfort after taking the supplement.

Glycerin

Often used as a solvent and/or preservative in liquids and to soften the gelatin used in softgels, glycerin can be derived from animals or plants. If you are vegetarian, make sure you look on the label to ensure it lists *vegetable* glycerin.

Gelatin

Derived from pig or cattle, gelatin is a common ingredient in both capsules and softgels. If the label lists gelatin, the supplement contains an animal product. Look for vegetarian or vegan capsules if this matters to you.

R℞ RX FROM DR. LOW DOG
Allergens and GMO

The Food Allergen Labeling and Consumer Protection Act (FAL-CPA), passed by Congress in August 2004, requires FDA-regulated packaged foods and dietary supplements to clearly state on the label when a food or product contains protein from one of the eight major allergens (milk, egg, peanuts, tree nuts, fish, shellfish, soy, and wheat). Please note that at the time of this writing, the list does not include corn. If you are sensitive to corn, watch for the words *vegetable coating* because such coatings are often made from corn. If you are vegan, have a milk allergy, or are lactose intolerant, watch for *lactose and lactate solids. Lactic acid may or may not be derived from dairy.* If you have celiac disease or are gluten sensitive, be cautious about brown rice syrup, which is often used in chewables and lozenges as an alternative to sugar. Brown rice syrup may be processed with barley enzymes, but whether these enzymes contain any residual barley gluten is not known.

People with celiac disease, gluten sensitivities, or corn allergies may be sensitive to maltodextrin, which comes from wheat, rice, potato, or corn. In the U.S., most companies use corn, while most in Europe use wheat. If the proteins have been removed during processing, and that's usually the case, you should be fine, but just keep this in mind.

Soybean oil is often used in both softgels and chewables. Only a small number of manufacturers insist on and can prove their soybean oil is not from genetically modified (non-GMO) soybeans. Also, most U.S. corn is genetically modified. Look for "organic" on the label to assure your product is non-GMO, as well as free of pesticides and harsh solvents.

Dyes and Preservatives

Some companies use natural colorings and flavorings in their products. Many cheaper supplements use artificial dyes to color their tablets, capsules, chewables or liquids, which I would generally avoid. Regulatory agencies in the U.S. and Europe consider titanium dioxide, used in food and supplements to give them a white appearance, an inert, nontoxic substance. You may have heard concerns about titanium dioxide, but these pertain primarily to nanoparticles used in cosmetics and sunscreens. The larger particles used in food and supplements do not present these same safety concerns.

There is ongoing debate about the effects of the synthetic FD&C colors on children's behavior, particularly yellow #5, red #40, or blue #2. These have also been linked to allergy-like reactions and possibly an adverse effect on the immune system. Increasingly, manufacturers are using vegetable dyes instead of synthetics. I generally tell my patients to avoid artificial colors and flavors, whether in food or supplements.

Some supplements use BHT (butylated hydroxytoluene) as an antioxidant and preservative. The Center for Science in the Public Interest puts BHT in its "caution" column, as some research suggests that it might be linked to cancer and/or disruption of the endocrine system. Granted, the amount you are getting in a once-daily multivitamin-mineral tablet would be small compared to what you would get from eating a bag of potato chips preserved with BHT. However, supplements can easily be made without it, so I'd avoid it.

Polysorbate 80, Croscarmellose Sodium, and Polyetheylene Glycol (PEG)

Polysorbate 80 is a natural sorbitol used in supplements to help make them more soluble. A 2005 toxicology study showed that it was safe at doses of 10 mg/kg body weight, that's far greater than what would be present in a tablet.

Croscarmellose sodium, also known as cross-linked sodium carboxymethyl cellulose or modified cellulose gum, is an ingredient that helps tablets break down in your stomach. Croscarmellose sodium is classified "generally recognized as safe" (GRAS) by the FDA, and after an extensive review of the safety data, the European Commission on Food Safety gave a green light for its safe use in dietary supplements.

Polyethylene glycol (PEG), made from petroleum gas or dehydration of alcohol, is used as a lubricating agent. Ingestion of large amounts have been shown to cause cancer and organ damage in animals. This is one I'd avoid.

10. SUGGESTED USE

The label may suggest when to take supplements, such as "Take one tablet twice daily with meals." I'll provide much more detailed information later in the book about when and how to take supplements for optimal benefits, as well as to prevent interference with medications.

11. CAUTIONS AND WARNINGS

The product may include a warning to alert consumers about certain precautions for using the product. If you are pregnant, breastfeeding, have a serious medical condition, or are taking prescription medications, it is especially important to pay attention to this section.

12. MANUFACTURER'S CONTACT INFORMATION

The law requires the manufacturer or distributor's place of business or phone number to appear on the label. This information is important if you ever want to contact a manufacturer to report a problem you had with their product (note that you will be asked for the lot number; see next item). You can also learn more details about the supplement by contacting the manufacturer or visiting their website.

13. LOT NUMBER

This is a series of numbers and/or letters that can be used to trace the product's manufacturing history. The lot number refers to a specific batch that was manufactured during a specific time period at a specific manufacturing facility. Lot numbers play a crucial role in the unlikely event of a product recall or in the case of a severe adverse event.

14. EXPIRATION DATE

This is the date when ingredients in the product will no longer have the full potency listed on the label. Sometimes, the date appears to run together with other numbers, so look carefully. To maximize shelf life, always store your supplements in a cool, dark cabinet. Oils (fish oil, flax oil) and probiotics should be kept in the refrigerator to prolong shelf life. Make sure to check expiration dates periodically and throw out any supplement that has expired.

15. QUALITY SEALS

A product may have a "seal" on its label, indicating it has passed an independent organization's quality assurance test. It means the product was properly manufactured, that it contains the ingredients listed on the label in the amount stated, and that it is free of harmful levels of contaminants. I strongly encourage you to choose manufacturers that use one of these quality labels. (Also see "Quality," page XX.)

I hope the labels are beginning to make more sense to you now. Now, let's dig a little deeper and talk about:

- Identifying nutritional gaps
- Determining the bioavailability and dissolution of supplements

- Being aware of potential interactions with other nutrients and medications
- Judging the overall quality of the supplements you are buying and using

I know that better understanding these topics will help you choose the right supplements for *you*.

RX FROM DR. LOW DOG

R An Important Equation:
RDA – Diet = Supplement

I always ask my patients to keep a food diary for two to three days to more accurately assess where their nutritional gaps are. To be sure you're getting the nutrients you need and not overdoing it, look at the RDA or AI for a specific nutrient, and then try to calculate what you are getting in your diet; supplement to make up the difference. Let's use calcium as an example: If you are 35 years old, you should be getting 1,000 mg every day. Estimate 300 mg for each serving of milk, yogurt, fortified nondairy milk, or cheese you eat most days. (Some cheese has 180 mg per serving, whereas some yogurts have 400 mg, so we'll just use 300 mg as your average dairy consumption per day.) Then add 250 mg, the amount of calcium you're getting from all other sources (cereal, leafy green vegetables) for the day. Let's assume that per day, your calcium from foods adds up as follows: 300 + 250 = 550 mg. Thus, you would need to increase your dietary intake and/or supplement with 450 mg of calcium to meet your 1,000 mg requirement. (*Note:* it's important to look at the label of a food to see how closely the serving size correlates to how much you are actually eating or drinking!)

BIOAVAILABILITY OF NUTRIENTS

Now that we've discussed what you will find on the dietary supplement label, it's time to turn our attention to how well you can digest, assimilate, and use the ingredients in these products. *Bioavailability* means that a nutrient or ingredient is absorbed in a form that is usable and able to reach the right target. For instance, if you are taking something to help your memory, you need to know that the nutrient will actually reach its target in the brain. Or if you're taking a supplement for your arthritic knees, will the ingredients reach the target? While many companies

RX FROM DR. LOW DOG

Home Test for Dissolution

Do you ever wonder whether your body is able to dissolve and absorb the vitamins you are taking? There's a home test that can answer your question.

To do the test, put the supplement tablet into a cup of hot, not boiling, water. Periodically stir the water, without touching the tablet, over a 30-minute period. By the end of the 30 minutes, your tablet should be pretty much disintegrated. If not, take it back to the store, ask for a refund, and buy a different brand.

Note: Tablets that are time-released, sustained-release, or enteric-coated would fail this dissolution test and that's okay. The first two products are designed to have a slower rate of disintegration, whereas enteric-coating is designed to minimize dissolution in the stomach.

advertise that their supplement is highly bioavailable, very few actually do testing to prove that claim is true.

Dissolution is the first step in bioavailability. Most reputable manufacturers ensure that their tablets will dissolve under normal conditions. If you are uncertain, do your own home test. Or choose capsules, softgels, liquids or powders, which have fewer issues with dissolution.

Besides dissolution, two other key factors affect bioavailability: whether your body recognizes the nutrient (a problem with some synthetic nutrients) and whether you have sufficient stomach acid and pancreatic enzymes to extract the nutrient from the supplement and absorb it into your bloodstream.

SYNTHETIC VERSUS NATURAL: DOES YOUR BODY KNOW THE DIFFERENCE?

One factor in the bioavailability of nutrients in supplements is whether they have the same molecular structure as the ones found in food. Many vitamins and minerals sold in the marketplace, as well as those found in fortified foods (cereals, milk, breads) are synthetic. Does it matter? It depends.

Generally speaking, the fat-soluble vitamins A, D, and E should be derived from natural sources whenever possible. Let's look at vitamin E as an example. Synthetic vitamin E is only half as biologically active as the natural form. Most foods fortified with vitamin E, as well as many supplements, use the synthetic form, which appears as dl-alpha tocopherol on the ingredients list. When purchasing a supplement, look for d-alpha tocopherol on the label, which indicates the natural form. There are actually eight forms of vitamin E (4 tocopherols and 4 tocotrienols), each with a unique function in the body. Using a mixture of tocopherols and tocotrienols might be the optimal way to supplement with vitamin E.

R̲X̲ RX FROM DR. LOW DOG
"Whole Food" Vitamins

Have you have ever seen a supplement claiming to be a "whole food" or "food-based" vitamin and wondered what it meant? In general, the terms are used to refer to vitamins that have undergone a fermenting process using yeast. It is thought that the assimilation and bioavailability of the vitamins is enhanced by taking advantage of the "biotransforming" nature of baker's or brewer's yeast *(Saccharomyces cerevisiae)*—an aspect of yeast that has long been exploited in the making of bread, wine, and ale.

These products are made by feeding vitamins (some natural, some synthetic) to yeast in a liquid broth solution. As the yeast grows, it incorporates the vitamins and minerals into its cellular structure. The yeast is then killed and dried, and the vitamins pressed into tablets or put into capsules, liquids, or powders. The theory is that the nutrients incorporated into the yeast are now in a highly bioavailable form. In some cases, such as chromium and selenium, science has shown this to be true. For other vitamins and minerals, it's unclear whether this is the case. On the label you will usually see ingredients listed as thiamine "derived from yeast" or "from *S. cerevisiae.*" Are these food-based or bio-transformed products worth the extra price? Many people think so as this is one of the fasting growing segments in the supplement industry. I personally take a multivitamin-mineral product made using this type of process.

In some cases, though, there is no difference between a synthetic and natural vitamin where the body is concerned. This is the case with vitamin C. If your supplement contains more than 100 mg of vitamin C, chances are high you're getting at least some synthetic vitamin C. However, natural and synthetic ascorbic acid are chemically identical and there are no known differences in their biological activities or bioavailability. Your body will be happy with either one and will use it effectively to perform all the tasks natural vitamin C would perform: boosting immunity, contributing to healthy gums, and so on.

DIGESTIVE JUICES: DO YOU HAVE ENOUGH?

Many nutrients in food or supplements require the presence of stomach acid and pancreatic enzymes. Stomach acids play a key role in helping the body use and absorb calcium, magnesium, iron, and B12. As we get older, we make less stomach acid, which is why people over the age of 50 should take a B12 supplement and/or eat foods fortified with B12. It's also why calcium citrate is recommended over carbonate, as it does not require stomach acid. Drugs that shut down stomach acid, such as PPIs, increase the risk for deficiencies of these nutrients. If you taking PPIs, make sure you are getting adequate amounts of these key nutrients. I discuss this more on page XXX in Appendix 4, "Drug-Nutrient Depletions and Interactions."

After leaving the stomach, food enters the small intestine where enzymes secreted by the pancreas further the digestion of proteins, carbohydrates, and particularly fats. Some people, such as those with cystic fibrosis, do not make enough pancreatic enzymes to digest and absorb the fat-soluble vitamins A, D, E and K, and are generally prescribed both pancreatic enzymes and supplements.

INTERACTIONS: SHOULD YOU BE CONCERNED?

Some nutrients can enhance or diminish the absorption of other nutrients. Large amounts of calcium (250 mg or more) can impair the absorption of iron, while vitamin C increases it. Interestingly, in the Southwest, people like to eat beans, which are high in iron, with chile (chili) peppers, which are packed with C. This traditional mixture maximized the absorption of plant-based iron, which is less absorbable than the iron found in meat. Iron supplements are best taken with food to avoid stomach upset. *Bottom line: If you take iron, take it with vitamin C, and not with large doses of calcium.*

Taking large doses of calcium or magnesium (250 mg or more) can compete with the absorption of other minerals, including each other, for absorption. I generally recommend taking magnesium at bedtime to help with sleep and relaxation. *Take your multiple vitamin-mineral supplement at least two hours apart from your calcium or magnesium.*

It is better to *take fat-soluble vitamins (A, D, E, K) and fish oil with a meal containing fat.* One study found that taking vitamin D with dinner instead of breakfast increased blood levels of vitamin D by about 50 percent!

Speaking of food, most vitamins and mineral supplements are best taken with food to aid their dissolution and absorption. *Multivitamin-mineral supplements* and *vitamins C, E, and B-complex can all be taken together at the same meal.* I recommend taking them with breakfast. Take larger amounts of calcium or magnesium several hours apart from other minerals. Calcium carbonate must be taken with food, whereas calcium citrate does not need to be. I recommend the latter.

There are a few supplements that should be taken on an empty stomach. Herbal bitters are often taken 20 minutes before a meal to "prime" the digestive tract, revving up the production of stomach acid and alerting the pancreas that food is coming. Bitter liqueurs, also known as digestifs, are common in Europe, where they are consumed as an evening cocktail before dinner to ensure healthy digestion! SAMe, a supplement used for mood problems, osteoarthritis, and fibromyalgia, is also recommended 20 to 30 minutes before a meal.

And what about medications? Certain nutrients can interact with the absorption and effectiveness of medications and vice versa. You will find information about the primary supplement-drug interactions and drug-induced nutrient depletions in Appendix 4, "Drug-Nutrient Depletions and Interactions." However, as a general rule: *Take your supplements two hours apart from any medicine.*

QUALITY

Dietary supplements should contain exactly what they say on the label—nothing more and nothing less. While the nutritional supplement industry as a whole has improved when it comes to quality control, there are still some major problem spots. As mentioned earlier, the worst offenders are products promoted for weight loss, sexual enhancement, and bodybuilding, as well as many supplement products coming from China and India.

Here are some unfortunate examples of how poor the quality of supplements can be. In 2010, researchers found that 14 of 20 dietary supplements marketed for weight loss were adulterated with prescription weight-loss drugs, and many contained sibutramine, a weight-loss drug withdrawn from the market because it increased the risk of heart attacks and strokes. A considerable number of sexual enhancement products labeled "all natural" have been found to contain prescription sildenafil (Viagra) and tadalafil (Cialis). Numerous traditional Chinese patent herbal medicines contain undeclared pharmaceutical drugs.

How can you identify companies that flout the law? For a start, trust common sense and your instincts. Supplements that claim to cure heart disease, cancer, or Alzheimer's are grossly overstating the science and preying upon people's fears and desperation. There is always going to be some exotic berry from the Amazon that "scientists have finally discovered" that manufacturers promote as having superpowers: It can make you lose weight, make your hair grow, and boost your sexual vigor . . . the list of claims is endless. If it sounds too good to be true, it probably is. Stay away from companies that trigger your natural skepticism.

Second, companies can convey to their customers that they are serious about quality by placing on their label a seal from an organization that certifies supplement quality. To use the seal, companies voluntarily submit to third party inspection of their manufacturing facility and independent testing of their products. If they pass these inspections and periodic testing of products, the product can include a quality seal on its label. When you purchase a product that bears one of these seals, you have reassurance that the product is made to high-quality standards. There are three primary organizations that offer these quality seals:

- **The United States Pharmacopeia:** As stated on its website, "The U.S. Pharmacopeial Convention (USP) is a scientific nonprofit organization that sets standards for the identity, strength, quality, and purity of medicines, food ingredients, and dietary supplements manufactured, distributed and consumed worldwide." The USP is an organization you can trust to provide top-notch scientific information—and the FDA enforces its drug standards in the U.S. (USP's standards are actually used by many countries.) I am proud to say that I served as the elected chair of the United States Pharmacopeia Dietary Supplements and Botanical Experts Information Committee for ten years before being elected and serving as chair of the Dietary Supplements and Botanicals Admissions Evaluation Subcommittee. Any company that follows the quality standards for a given dietary supplement published in the United States Pharmacopeia can put the letters "USP" after the ingredient—just like when you buy a generic aspirin and it says acetylsalicylic acid USP. That means it follows all the quality control and manufacturing steps set by the USP. While drug companies are required by law to follow these guidelines, unfortunately dietary supplement manufacturers are not. See *www.usp.org/usp-verification-services/usp-verified-dietary-supplements*.

- **NSF International:** The NSF (formerly the National Sanitation Foundation) is an independent organization of scientists and public health experts that sets standards for supplements and tests and certifies them. This is a highly rigorous program and any company that bears the seal is of superior quality. See *http://info.nsf.org/Certified/Dietary/*.
- **Consumer Labs** is a private company that tests numerous branded products and allows companies that pass its quality tests to use its seal. Consumer Labs also offers testing information to the public via a subscription. This can be a great way to see whether your brand of supplements passes muster! See *http://www.consumerlab.com/seal.asp*.

If you would like to know more about the safety and quality of supplements, and the research behind them, there are several excellent websites you can check. See the Resources section at the rear of this book and also Chapter 7, where I talk in more detail about science and research in the field of nutritional supplements.

Despite the abundance of information that gets crowded onto a tiny label and wrapped around a little jar, I hope now you feel you are a more educated consumer of nutritional supplements. Now it's time to turn our attention to one of the most important categories of nutrients: vitamins.

Chapter 3

Vitamins

I vividly remember the taste of cod liver oil when I was little. One word: yuck! I'm not sure my mom knew that cod liver oil was such as excellent source of vitamins A and D, and omega-3 fatty acids, providing vital nourishment for our eyes, skin, brain, bones, and immune system. She just knew it was good for children! And while I didn't appreciate it then, I certainly do now.

Vitamins are critically important to your health. You need sufficient amounts not only to stave off disease but more importantly, to promote vitality and well-being. Yet you also don't want to overdo it. Take the Goldilocks approach: Aim for an amount that's not too high or too low, but just right.

As you read through this chapter, you might find that there are key vitamins that you might be deficient in due to age, medication use, or a specific health issue. If you think you might be lacking, you might want to consider getting some laboratory tests done that can provide your actual levels. If you don't want to have laboratory testing done, keep a two-day food diary (you'll find a form on page XX) and then use the resources provided at the end of this book to determine whether you are getting enough of key nutrients.

Personally, I believe that the best way to ensure you're getting all your essential vitamins is to take a basic multivitamin-mineral supplement if you're not doing so already. If you stay within the ranges I provide in this chapter, it's highly unlikely that you are going to get too much of any vitamin. Because some medications deplete vitamins and other nutrients, and some nutrients alter the effectiveness of certain medications, be sure to check out Appendix 4, "Drug-Nutrient Depletions and Interactions."

In this chapter, I've included information about each vitamin, food sources, signs of deficiency, who is at risk for deficiency, the recommended daily allowance (RDA) or adequate intake (AI), the daily value (DV), the tolerable upper limit (UL), and any specifics you should be aware of when reviewing the dietary supplement label. If you have vitamin bottles at home, now would be a good time to take them out and see how they compare to what is listed here. Let's look at vitamins A through K and get a little more familiar with what they are and why they are so necessary for your health.

VITAMIN A

In the ancient medical scrolls of Egypt, liver was recommended for the treatment of night blindness. During the 13th century, Jacob van Maerlandt, a Dutch physician, wrote the following:

> *Who does not at night see right*
> *Eats the liver of the goat*
> *He will then see better at night*

However, it wasn't until the 1920s that the fat-soluble compound in liver that plays such a vital role in sight was isolated and named vitamin A. And as you will soon see, vitamin A is responsible for far more than just seeing well in the darkness.

Vitamin A is a group of fat-soluble vitamins that come in two primary forms: animal-derived and plant-derived. Animal-derived vitamin A is referred to as retinol, or *pre*formed vitamin A, and is the most biologically active form. Some plant-derived vitamin A, especially the colorful carotenoids in fruits and vegetables, can be converted when needed to the active, or retinol form of vitamin A. Thus, these carotenoids are referred to as "*pro*vitamin A." Roughly 70 to 90 percent of the body's vitamin A is stored in the liver, which is why eating liver provides such a whopping amount of the nutrient.

WHAT IT DOES: Notice the similarity between the words *retinol* and *retina?* Retinol is carried in the bloodstream to the retina in the back of the eye, where it's stored and used to help us see in low levels of light. While the ancients did not know about vitamins, they were astute in their observation that eating liver could help treat night blindness. As vitamin A levels fall in the body, it becomes increasingly difficult to see in dim light. This is because it plays a key role in the formation of rhodopsin, the visual pigment in the retina that is essential for the eyes to adapt to the dark.

Vitamin A maintains the health of the cells that line our nose, throat, and respiratory, digestive, and urinary tracts. This barrier serves as our body's first line of defense against infection. If a microbe should get past the barrier, vitamin A helps activate our immune cells so that we can fight the infection. In the bones, retinol is needed to produce red blood cells and for helping integrate iron into hemoglobin so the blood can carry oxygen to all the tissues in our body. Vitamin A is important for the proper expression of our genes and is necessary during pregnancy for ensuring the healthy formation of the baby's heart, eyes, ears, arms, and legs.

You may have seen retinol in topical creams designed to reduce wrinkles. Its antioxidant activity penetrates into the deep layers of collagen that provide support for the skin. While that all sounds good, in 2012 the National Toxicology Program found that when retinyl palmitate and retinoic acid are applied topically, they accelerate the growth of skin cancers upon exposure to sun. This is very concerning. I recommend you avoid using topical retinol preparations or, if you really feel you must use them, apply only at night when you won't be exposed to the sun.

FOOD SOURCES: Preformed vitamin A is found in a number of animal-based foods. Three ounces of beef liver provides almost ten times the RDA for women, while three ounces of chicken liver provides roughly double. Foods that provide between 10 and 30 percent of the RDA include shrimp, eggs, whole milk, yogurt, butter, and cheese. In the United States, we also fortify cereals, breads, low-fat/skim milk, and infant formula with *synthetic* preformed vitamin A.

Carotenoids are found in carrots, pumpkin, apricots, broccoli, and dark green leafy vegetables, such as spinach. Only a few of the dietary carotenoids—beta-carotene, and beta-cryptoxanthin—can be readily converted into retinol. Lycopene, lutein, and zeaxanthin are also carotenoids but have no vitamin A activity.

To enhance the absorption of carotenoids in food, you *must* take them with some fat. This is really important! Beta-carotene in oil has about half the activity of preformed vitamin A, and without oil, it has just one-sixth of the activity! I cook spinach over low heat with a little butter and fresh garlic and I roast butternut squash with olive oil, cinnamon, and a pinch of salt. When you gently heat the food, the carotenoids are released into the oil or fat, increasing absorption. If you are taking beta-carotene in a supplement, take it with a fat-containing meal.

SIGNS OF DEFICIENCY: A condition known as xerophthalmia, or extreme dryness of the eyes, is often one of the first signs of vitamin A deficiency. It can lead to blindness if left untreated. Other signs include dry, scaly skin and frequent diarrhea and respiratory infections, particularly in children.

RISK FOR DEFICIENCY: Globally, those at risk for deficiency are primarily pregnant and breastfeeding women, newborns, and children. Tragically, 100 to 140 million children around the world are vitamin A deficient and 300,000 to 500,000 will go blind every year as a result. Since vitamin A is also vitally important for our immune defense, many of these children die from respiratory infections and diarrhea. In the U.S., vitamin A deficiency is primarily found in those who are malnourished, alcoholics, take certain medications, or have cystic fibrosis, Crohn's disease, ulcerative colitis, or pancreatic insufficiency.

RDA/AI: Men: 3,000 IU
Women: 2,333 IU
Pregnant: 2,567 IU
Breastfeeding: 4,333 IU

DV: 5,000 IU

UL: 10,000 IU per day. The primary concern is getting too much *preformed* vitamin A. This can be particularly dangerous during pregnancy. More than 10,000 IU per day can cause a miscarriage or birth defects in the baby. There are numerous vitamin A supplements and multivitamins in the marketplace that contain 10,000 IU or even higher levels, of preformed vitamin A. A number of prescription drugs used to treat acne (e.g., isotretinoin [Accutane]) and psoriasis (acitretin [Soriatane]), contain synthetic forms of retinol. These medications can be very dangerous in pregnancy. If a fertile woman is taking them, she must use appropriate birth control measures. You should NOT take supplements containing retinol if you are taking one of these drugs.

The body only converts the provitamin A carotenoids to the active retinol form of vitamin A when needed. Studies of high-dose long-term beta-carotene supplements have failed to show that they increase serum retinol above normal levels. Other than some reports of a temporary yellowing of the skin, no serious side effects have been reported with long-term administration of high doses of beta-carotene—with *one important exception*. A review of four studies (109,394 subjects) found that when current, but not former, smokers and people who had been exposed to asbestos were given high-dose beta-carotene supplements (33,000–50,000 IU per day), lung cancer risk increased by 24 percent. So, if you smoke, stop! And meanwhile, to be on the safe side, make sure your multivitamin doesn't contain more than 2,500 IU of beta-carotene.

SUPPLEMENT CONSIDERATIONS: *For overall health,* take a multivitamin that provides 5,000 IU of vitamin A with no more than 50 percent as preformed vitamin A (2,500 IU) and the balance as beta-carotene and/or mixed carotenoids. Natural preformed vitamin A is usually listed on the label as retinyl acetate, retinol acetate, or vitamin A acetate.

Retinyl palmitate or vitamin A palmitate is usually synthetic and is the form used in fortified foods and in some supplements. It is also perfectly fine to take a multivitamin that contains all of its vitamin A as beta-carotene and/or mixed carotenoids, which is what I do.

Smokers: Do *not* purchase supplements that provide more than 2,500 IU of beta-carotene.

People who regularly eat liver (3-4 times per month) or take cod liver oil should *not* take supplements containing preformed vitamin A. Choose supplements that provide vitamin A as beta-carotene or mixed carotenoids.

That brings me back to the cod liver oil I was given as a child. It's really important to read the label to know how much vitamin A it contains because you don't want to be taking cod liver oil that provides 4,000 IU preformed vitamin A per teaspoon *and* a multivitamin that provides 5,000 IU preformed vitamin A. When you add what you are getting in your diet, you can easily go over the UL. I take a high-quality Norwegian cod liver oil that provides 850 IU per day of preformed vitamin A, as well as 400 IU of vitamin D3 *and* 1,100 mg of marine omega-3 fatty acids. I take cod liver oil because I prefer preformed vitamin A in its most natural form. Because I use cod liver oil, I take a multivitamin that contains 100 percent of the vitamin A as mixed carotenoids.

PARTNER NUTRIENTS: Zinc is absolutely necessary for transporting the retinol stored in the liver to where it needs to go, such as your eyes. Vitamin A makes a nice partner for iron as it helps move the iron into hemoglobin. Taking vitamin A and iron, along with vitamin C, is often the best way to correct iron deficiency anemia. Beta-carotene improves the absorption of lycopene, which is particularly beneficial for the prostate.

SPECIAL POPULATIONS: We all need vitamin A, but going over the UL can be a problem—and it's especially dangerous for pregnant women. The best way to ensure you get enough vitamin A without exceeding the UL is to eat a diet rich in vitamin A from plant and animal sources. Prenatal vitamins should contain no more than 3,000 IU of preformed vitamin A (the RDA for pregnant women).

RX FROM DR. LOW DOG
Preformed Vitamin A and Bone Health

In the early 2000s, studies published in the *Journal of the American Medical Association* and the *New England Journal of Medicine* suggested that prolonged intake of 5,000 IU per day of preformed vitamin A could increase the risk of brittle bones and fracture. However, several recent studies have found that high doses of preformed vitamin A (up to 25,000 IU per day) taken over many years did not have a negative impact on bone. That's reassuring, but there is *no* reason to take this much vitamin A without the guidance of a qualified health professional. If your multivitamin provides very high doses of preformed vitamin A, find another one.

B-VITAMINS

The B-vitamins are water-soluble vitamins that have a similar function, even though molecularly they are each quite unique. Did you ever wonder how they got their numbers and why there isn't a B4, B8 or B11? Well, it turns out that thiamine gets the distinct pleasure of being number 1 (B1) because it was the first B-vitamin identified; it was isolated in 1910. When riboflavin was discovered in 1920, it had similar functions to thiamine and so was named B2. The reason there are gaps between the numbers are because these slots were originally taken up by substances thought to be vitamins that later turned out not to be, so they were removed from the list. And to further complicate things, even though vitamin B12 was discovered before B3, we didn't know that it functioned like other B-vitamins until much later, hence its number!

Because the B-vitamins have similar functions, they work synergistically together. For example vitamins B6, B9, and B12 work together to protect our cardiovascular and nervous systems. Multivitamins and B-complex vitamins generally contain all eight of the B-vitamins. You can also purchase individual B-vitamins if you have specific issues you are trying to address.

B-vitamins are often referred to as "stress vitamins" for good reason. The B-vitamins not only play important roles in the metabolism of carbohydrates, fats, and proteins and in the production of fuel and energy, but they are crucial for the production of brain chemicals that help to regulate our mood, sleep, and feeling of pleasure. Given the incredible stress many people are living under, I believe the B-vitamins are incredibly important.

I strongly recommend supplementation for: women who are pregnant or planning to be (folate), or anyone who has diabetes (B-complex), drinks heavily (B-complex and thiamine particularly), is vegan (vitamin B12), takes PPI or metformin medications (vitamin B12), is under considerable emotional or physical stress (B-complex), or has problems with memory or heart disease (B-complex).

Now let's take a deeper look at each one of these very important vitamins.

VITAMIN B1 (THIAMINE)

More than 1,300 years ago, Chinese physicians observed that a considerable number of people living in southern China suffered from a condition marked by swelling of the legs and/or severe weakness and tingling in the feet. This condition was not seen in people living in northern China. These physicians were describing beriberi, a disease caused by thiamine deficiency. Although they did not know the cause of this ailment, they suspected it had something to do with the fact that people in southern China ate lots of polished rice, while those in the north consumed wheat. They found that giving people remedies containing rice polishings and millet bran improved the condition. Both are sources of thiamine. Today we know that excessive refining and polishing of rice removes considerable proportions of B-vitamins.

Although beriberi is not common in the United States, many of us have marginal levels of this important water-soluble vitamin. Very little thiamine is stored in the body and depletion can be rapid, occurring in as little as two weeks! This means it must constantly be replenished.

WHAT IT DOES: Thiamine plays a vital role in your body's production of energy. It is a coenzyme, or helper nutrient—for enzymes that are responsible for the converting food to energy, particularly the metabolism of carbohydrates, glucose, and alcohol. Because we consume so many sugar-laden, nutrient devoid carbohydrates, we require a constant supply of thiamine. Diabetics are in particular need of thiamine. Studies show that it can help prevent or slow the development of diabetes related complications of the cardiovascular system, kidneys, and eyes.

Thiamine is vital for the healthy function of our brain, as well as our nervous and cardiovascular systems. Research suggests this vitamin plays a vital role in helping our body deal with stress and preserving our memory as we age. Some, though not all, studies show it may be beneficial for those with dementia. Two small studies found that compared to placebo, thiamine improves heart function in those with heart failure. Thiamine may also help prevent cataracts. Although you may have heard that thiamine helps prevent mosquito bites, the research shows that's probably more fiction than fact!

FOOD SOURCES: Pork, trout, macadamia nuts, sunflower seeds, green peas, acorn squash, asparagus, oatmeal, beans, flaxseeds, brown rice, and yeast are good sources of natural thiamine. In the U.S., cereal grains are fortified with thiamine, providing anywhere from 25 to 100 percent of your daily needs.

SIGNS OF DEFICIENCY: Thiamine deficiency impacts multiple systems in the body: neurological, cardiovascular, gastrointestinal, and musculoskeletal. Early signs of deficiency include loss of appetite, constipation, irritability, and depression. As the severity and duration of the deficiency increases, symptoms worsen.

Three conditions are caused by severe thiamine deficiency: beriberi, Wernicke encephalopathy, and Wernicke-Korsakoff syndrome. Beriberi can cause neurological symptoms, such as muscle weakness, tingling in the legs, difficulty speaking, vomiting, mental confusion, and strange eye movements (nystagmus), and/or cardiovascular symptoms—rapid heartbeat, water retention, enlarged heart, or even heart failure. Wernicke encephalopathy damages the lower parts of the brain and leads to poor muscle control, nystagmus, and mental confusion. Wernicke-Korsakoff psychosis happens when the parts of the brain involved with memory are permanently damaged. People are unable to form any new memories and often suffer the loss of old memories, as well. Wernicke-Korsakoff is most often seen in alcoholics and those who are severely malnourished. While on my neurology rotation during medical school, our team admitted to the hospital a woman who was homeless and an alcoholic after the police found her staggering and incoherent. In spite of our giving her thiamine and other important nutrients, her short-term memory never returned. It was heartbreaking.

RISK FOR DEFICIENCY: Borderline thiamine deficiency may be more common than we realize because we consume large quantities of carbohydrates that require thiamine for their metabolism. Diabetics often develop deficiency over time, because thiamine is required for the enzymes involved in the metabolism of glucose. Excess carbohydrates, diabetes, and obesity all go hand in hand, which is why obesity is often associated with thiamine deficiency. One study of obese patients who were preparing to undergo bariatric surgery found that 29 percent were deficient in thiamine. Another study of 378 adults found that thiamine deficiency was highest in obese Hispanics (47 percent) and African Americans (31 percent), compared to obese Caucasians (7 percent).

Alcoholics are at very high risk for deficiency. In fact, up to 80 percent of heavy drinkers have some degree of thiamine deficiency because to metabolize alcohol, the body needs thiamine, yet alcohol impairs absorption of thiamine from the intestinal tract. People with *chronic liver disease* may also require supplementation.

People who have had bariatric (weight-loss) surgery are at risk for deficiency. In fact, almost one in five people develop thiamine deficiency after undergoing gastric bypass.

People with severe morning sickness or any other condition associated with frequent vomiting (such as bulimia), can develop thiamine deficiency.

Anyone who regularly eats raw fish and shellfish could become thiamine deficient because these foods contain thiaminase, an enzyme that makes thiamine unusable by the body. Cooking destroys thiaminase, so eating cooked fish and seafood is fine.

Coffee and tea drinkers who are low in vitamin C should be wary. Coffee and tea, even decaf, contain antithiamine factors, which can prevent thiamine from being absorbed. This is generally only a problem if you consume large amounts (5–6 cups per day) and you are low in vitamin C.

RDA/AI: Men: 1.2 mg   Women: 1.1 mg
Pregnancy: 1.4 mg
Breastfeeding: 1.4 mg

DV: 1.5 mg

UL: None. No serious adverse effects have been noted with long-term oral supplementation of up to 200 mg per day. When high doses of thiamine are consumed, the excess is rapidly excreted in the urine.

SUPPLEMENT CONSIDERATIONS: A multivitamin that provides 1.5 to 3.0 mg per day is adequate for most of us, but aim for 10 to 30 mg per day if you have diabetes or are taking thiamine-depleting medications. Drinking two or more servings of alcohol per day? Take 25 to 50 mg of thiamine to protect your brain and nervous system. If you have heart failure or kidney disease, ask your health-care provider to check your thiamine levels. You may need much higher doses.

Most thiamine in supplements and fortified foods is synthetic and referred to as thiamine mononitrate or thiamine hydrochloride on the label. Benfotiamine is a fat-soluble form of thiamine shown to be highly effective for restoring low thiamine levels. The dose is typically 150 to 300 mg taken one or two times per day with food until thiamine levels are normalized.

PARTNER NUTRIENTS: B-vitamins are best taken together in a complex. Thiamine is highly dependent on magnesium, so make sure you are getting an adequate supply of both. Diabetics and people with heart disease are often low in both thiamine and magnesium, which is double trouble. If you love coffee and/or tea, make sure you're getting adequate amounts of vitamin C, as it blocks the antithiamine effects of these beverages.

SPECIAL POPULATIONS: Thiamine is important for the body's production of energy, so people who are highly athletic or have physically demanding jobs may require additional thiamine. Pregnant and breastfeeding mothers require additional amounts to support energy production, too—as do adolescents when they are going through their growth spurts.

VITAMIN B2 (RIBOFLAVIN)

In 1879, researchers identified a yellow-green colored compound in milk whey that they named lactoflavin (*lacto* for milk and *flavin* from the Latin *flavus*, or "yellow"). In 1933, this same yellow, water-soluble substance was isolated from yeast and given the name riboflavin. The name derives from the word *ribose*, a type of sugar that is part of this vitamin's molecular structure, and *flavin*, as mentioned previously. When riboflavin (vitamin B2) is taken as a supplement, it is what gives the urine a harmless strong yellow-orange discoloration.

WHAT IT DOES: Riboflavin serves as a helper, or co-factor, in many enzyme reactions that are involved in the body's production of energy. It maintains the health of our nervous system and eyes, helps us break down and use dietary proteins and fats, and converts vitamins B6 and B9 (folate) to their active forms in the body. Riboflavin plays an important role in the maintenance of our 24-hour circadian rhythm by activating blue light–sensitive cells in the retina, inhibiting the production of melatonin (a hormone that signals the body to let it know it's time to sleep). A 2015 study published by researchers at the National Eye Institute in the journal *Ophthalmology* found that high dietary intakes of riboflavin are highly protective against cataracts.

Riboflavin has been studied for the prevention of migraine headaches. A current theory is that migraines are caused by mitochrondrial dysfunction in brain cells. (Mitochondria are the powerhouses within our cells.) Riboflavin helps maintain normal energy production in brain mitochondria. At a dose of 400 mg per day, riboflavin is "strongly recommended" for migraine prophylaxis according to the Canadian Headache Society guidelines and receives a "probably effective" rating from the American Academy of Neurology and American Headache Society.

Riboflavin, with the help of vitamin C, increases the level of glutathione, one of our body's most potent antioxidants. Riboflavin is vitally important for maintaining the health of our cells, providing energy to the body and maintaining a healthy immune system. Some evidence even suggests that riboflavin has anticancer properties, particularly for colorectal cancer and possibly cervical cancer, as well.

Riboflavin is crucial for the absorption and use of iron in the body. Studies in the United Kingdom using laboratory data, not just dietary questionnaires, found that adolescent girls were at significantly high risk for riboflavin deficiency. Interestingly, teenage girls are also at high risk for iron deficiency anemia. Recently, a five-year study of more than 1,200 people in China found a strong correlation between low riboflavin and iron and concluded that "correcting inadequate riboflavin intake may be a priority in the prevention of anemia."

FOOD SOURCES: In many countries, milk and dairy are the primary sources of riboflavin in the diet. Meat, particularly beef liver, and fatty fish are also excellent sources. Good sources of riboflavin can be found in green vegetables, such as broccoli and Brussels sprouts, mushrooms, nuts, eggs, soybeans, brewer's yeast, and whole grains. Refined grain products are fortified in the U.S. because riboflavin is typically lost during processing. Riboflavin is heat stable and not damaged during cooking. However, it is degraded by light, which is why dairy and grains should be stored in dark containers.

SIGNS OF DEFICIENCY: As riboflavin levels fall, people may begin to exhibit mild signs of deficiency within just a couple of weeks. They initially will experience low energy and insomnia, and the eyes begin to fatigue easily, becoming increasingly sensitive to light. The skin is affected: The scalp, ears, eyelids, and genital area may begin to itch and scale, the corners of the mouth may begin to crack. Some people experience sore throat and lowered immunity. The tongue may take on a magenta colored appearance. Anemia may develop if riboflavin deficiency is prolonged.

RISK FOR DEFICIENCY: Riboflavin deficiency, called ariboflavinosis, is commonly seen in populations that do not consume dairy or meat. A study of Swedish vegans found that over 90 percent were not getting enough riboflavin in their diet. Riboflavin deficiency is more common in teenagers, especially girls, and among elders on restricted diets. Alcoholics are also at high risk for deficiency.

RDA/AI: Men: 1.3 mg   Women: 1.1 mg

Pregnancy: 1.4 mg

Breastfeeding: 1.6 mg

DV: 1.7 mg

UL: ND. Riboflavin toxicity is generally not a problem because of limited intestinal absorption. Doses of 400 mg per day have been used to prevent migraine headaches and are well tolerated.

SUPPLEMENT CONSIDERATIONS: Riboflavin and riboflavin 5'-monophosphate are the two most common forms found in dietary supplements.

PARTNER NUTRIENTS: Riboflavin partners with the other B-vitamins. Riboflavin is needed to activate vitamin B6 (pyridoxine) and B9 (folate), and is necessary for converting tryptophan to niacin. Riboflavin is necessary for the absorption and use of iron.

SPECIAL POPULATIONS: Diabetics can have low riboflavin as they excrete higher levels in their urine and should definitely supplement with 3 to 5 mg of this important B-vitamin. If you are at risk for cataracts, I encourage you to take a daily multivitamin that contains 3 to 5 mg of riboflavin. Teenage girls would benefit from a basic multivitamin-mineral supplement that provides at least the DV for riboflavin, as well as iron. Athletes should also ensure that they are getting adequate amounts of B2 through food and supplementation. Those suffering from migraines might want to consider a trial of riboflavin. If you have elevated homocysteine levels (a condition that prevents the body from converting this chemical into methionine, an amino acid needed for breaking down fats and involved in many metabolic functions), taking riboflavin, along with vitamins B6, B9, and B12, should be considered.

VITAMIN B3 (NIACIN)

During the first 40 years of the 20th century, a strange but deadly disease took the lives of tens of thousands of poor people in the United States. People lost their hair, developed extreme sensitivity to the sun that caused a terrible red scaling of the skin, had persistent diarrhea; became weak and aggressive, and developed mental confusion or dementia before they died. No one knew what was responsible. There had been reports of a similar mystery disease in Europe in the mid- to late 19th century, thought to be due to some type of infection.

It took a lot of detective work to discover that a new world plant, corn, was at the center of this unknown illness. Corn had been brought from the Americas to Europe and then spread to Africa and Asia. From 1750 to 1850, it became a staple in the typical peasant's diet, which was generally low in meat, eggs, and dairy. France, Italy, and Egypt suffered massive epidemics of the condition I described. They named it pellagra, from the Italian words *pelle agra,* meaning "rough skin," in reference to the skin sores and rashes. Meanwhile, in the late 1800s, Americans began to eat high amounts of processed corn, and cornmeal became heavily integrated into the diets of poor southerners, who also ate few animal products.

In 1923, a public health officer by the name of Joseph Goldberger solved the mystery: Pellagra was a nutritional disease that could be corrected with dried brewer's yeast, milk, meat, or eggs. Brewer's yeast contains readily bioavailable niacin, and because only a small amount was needed to prevent or reverse pellagra, it became the treatment of choice. Over the next 20 years, bakers began voluntarily fortifying their flour with brewer's or baker's yeast, and states started requiring the enrichment of wheat flour, cornmeal, and grits. The effects were dramatic. The pellagra rate in Mississippi dropped from 101 per 100,000 in 1946 to 1 per 100,000 in 1947. To date, pellagra is the most severe nutritional deficiency disease in American history.

But why was corn such a problem? There were many poor people living in what is now the southwestern United States, Mexico, and Central America who relied on corn as a dietary staple but did not suffer from pellagra. That's because the Aztecs, Maya, Hopi, and other indigenous peoples prepared their corn by a process known as nixtamalization, a multistep process that entailed soaking, cooking, and steeping the corn in a lime or alkali solution prior to its being washed, hulled, and ground. This freed the niacin in the corn, making it bioavailable. Unfortunately, this practice was not adopted by the peoples in Europe, Africa, and Asia, or by the large industrial American mills. They didn't know that it was critically important for the nutritional value of corn. This process is still in use by some companies today, which is why you see "corn treated with lime" or "*maíz nixtamalizado*" (the phrase in Spanish) on packages of corn tortillas.

The other key part of this story was that poor people relying on improperly prepared corn also had diets lacking in animal products, which are readily available sources of the amino acid tryptophan. It turns out that the body can make niacin out of tryptophan if necessary. If people had been eating corn with cheese, eggs, chicken, beef, or beans, they probably would have avoided pellagra.

WHAT IT DOES: Niacin (also known as nicotinic acid) and niacinamide (also called nicotinamide) are two forms of vitamin B3, a water-soluble vitamin. Niacin is a major player in converting carbohydrates, proteins, and fats into fuel. It promotes cellular health and protects our DNA from damage, and research shows that niacin protects against oral and esophageal cancers. A study of airline pilots, who are subject to high exposures of radiation, found that niacin, but not other antioxidants, reduced DNA damage. Niacin, both orally and topically, also seems to offer some protection against skin cancer.

Before we had statins, niacin was the drug of choice for treating cholesterol problems. Doses in the range of 2,000 to 3,000 mg per day on average increased HDL cholesterol by 30 percent, decreased LDL cholesterol by 21 percent, and lowered triglycerides by 44 percent—impressive! But we know that heart disease involves more than just your cholesterol and triglycerides levels (your lipid profile). Two recent large studies found that while niacin improved lipid profiles, it did not reduce heart attacks or save lives. Statin medications were shown to do both, which is why today niacin is mainly prescribed for those individuals who are at high risk for heart disease but can't tolerate statins. Make sure you talk to your health-care provider *before* using high-dose niacin for managing your cholesterol and/or triglycerides. These doses require close follow-up to ensure there is no damage to the liver.

One of the symptoms of niacin deficiency is dementia, so there has been interest in looking at its potential role in Alzheimer's. Preliminary research shows that people who eat niacin-rich foods and/or get niacin in their multivitamins (17–45 mg/day) have a lower risk of developing Alzheimer's disease than those who consume less than 14 mg/day of niacin.

Some studies also show that along with other nutrients such as beta-carotene, zinc, and lutein, niacin may help prevent or slow the progression of age-related macular degeneration, as well as prevent cataracts.

Although niacinamide (nicotinamide) does not lower cholesterol like niacin does, researchers found that it reduces the pain and increases the flexibility of arthritic joints. Dermatologists also use topical niacinamide for treating eczema, acne, and rosacea. Studies show that when applied topically, it reduces puffiness and blotchiness, decreases fine lines and wrinkles, and reduces areas of hyperpigmentation ("age spots"). Don't be surprised to find this vitamin increasingly being used in moisturizers and antiwrinkle creams!

FOOD SOURCES: Niacin is naturally found in meat, poultry, brewer's yeast, beef liver, salmon, tuna, sunflower seeds, beans, and peanuts. Bread and cereals are usually fortified with niacin, often providing 25 percent of the DV. The body can also make niacin from the amino acid tryptophan, which is readily found in poultry, beef, eggs, beans, and dairy products.

SIGNS OF DEFICIENCY: Heartburn, abdominal bloating, mouth sores, and constipation can occur during the early stages of niacin deficiency. With prolonged deficiency, the tongue and mouth become red and swollen; a thick, scaly rash develops on skin exposed to sunlight; nausea, vomiting, diarrhea, fatigue, depression, disorientation, and cognitive decline can all occur. In medical school I was taught to remember pellagra by the three Ds: dermatitis (scaly rash on skin after exposure to sunlight), diarrhea, and dementia (disorientation, cognitive decline).

RISK FOR DEFICIENCY: Thanks to food fortification programs, significant niacin deficiency is not common in Western populations. However, mild forms of niacin deficiency may be more prevalent than we realize, especially in alcoholics, those with absorption problems, the homeless or malnourished, and people with cancer. Hartnup's disease causes poor absorption of tryptophan, which can also put patients at risk for niacin deficiency. People with carcinoid syndrome use up all their tryptophan making serotonin and could also become niacin deficient.

RDA/AI: Men: 16 mg Women: 14 mg
Pregnancy: 18 mg
Breastfeeding: 17 mg

DV: 20 mg

UL: 35 mg

Note: 2–3 grams per day is often used to treat high cholesterol, but this should only be done under the supervision of a health-care professional.

SUPPLEMENT CONSIDERATIONS: A multivitamin that provides 20 to 30 mg per day of niacin or niacinamide is sufficient for most of us. However, reading the label can sometimes be a challenge. Niacin, also listed on the label as nicotinic acid, is available in "immediate-release," "slow-release," and "timed-release" forms. Some people use the time-released form of niacin because it is less likely than the immediate-release form to cause flushing at doses greater than 200 mg. Flushing involves not just a rush of blood to the face but tingling, itching, and burning in the face, arms, and chest, all of which can be kind of scary! This is why people taking high-dose niacin for cholesterol are often told to take one 325 mg aspirin 30 minutes before their niacin to prevent flushing.

Prolonged use of high-dose niacin may cause glucose intolerance, liver damage, and gastrointestinal distress. And while timed-release niacin may reduce flushing, it is much more likely to be harmful to your liver. If you are taking more than 500 mg of niacin in a dietary supplement, please make sure that your health-care provider is aware of this and is periodically checking your liver enzymes.

Instead of taking nicotinic acid, you might want to use niacinamide, the form of niacin found in many dietary supplements and fortified foods. On the label, it can also be listed as nicotinamide, NAD, NADP, or NADH. Niacinamide does not cause flushing and is much safer in larger doses than niacin or nicotinic acid. However, this form is not useful for treating cholesterol/lipid problems.

PARTNER NUTRIENTS: All the B-vitamins work better when taken together, but niacin absolutely requires vitamin B6 as a partner.

SPECIAL POPULATIONS: Diabetics should note that taking high doses of niacin (the amount used to lower cholesterol) might increase blood sugar levels. People who are exposed to higher levels of UV radiation, such as pilots or those at risk for skin cancer, should ensure that they are getting at least the DV of niacin.

PANTOTHENIC ACID (VITAMIN B5)

Pantothenic acid, vitamin B5—a water-soluble member of the B-complex family—takes its name from the Greek *pantothen,* which means "on all sides," because small quantities of this vitamin are found in nearly every food, making deficiency in humans exceedingly rare.

WHAT IT DOES: Pantothenic acid plays a vital role in the metabolism of carbohydrates and fats, assisting in the production and storage of energy in the body. It is a primary component of coenzyme A (CoA), a helper or cofactor for more than 70 different enzymatic pathways in the body, including the production of acetylcholine, a neurotransmitter involved in memory, learning, attention, and the contraction of skeletal muscles. CoA is also involved in the production of melatonin, antibodies, adrenal hormones, and heme, the protein in hemoglobin that carries oxygen throughout the body. Pantethine, the stable form of pantothenic acid, has been shown in some small studies to mildly improve cholesterol levels and the ability of blood to clot, though I would not rely on it for the Many shampoos contain panthenol, chemically similar to pantothenic acid, because it acts as a lubricant, improving the appearance and texture of hair. When used in moisturizing creams, it softens skin. While some companies claim that pantothenic acid in shampoo can delay the graying of hair, there is no evidence that it does. Studies show that pantothenol can aid in wound healing when applied topically.

FOOD SOURCES: Pantothenic acid is abundant in shiitake mushrooms (richest source), avocados (second richest source), organ meats, brewer's yeast, eggs, beans, chicken, broccoli, mushrooms, and sweet potatoes. Whole grains are another good source. However, refining grains causes a dramatic loss of this vitamin, as does the canning of many foods. Intestinal bacteria can produce pantothenic acid, but we don't know whether or not it is then absorbed and used by the body.

SIGNS OF DEFICIENCY: We have very few examples of pantothenic acid deficiency, but signs and symptoms noted in voluntary deficiency studies and in prisoners of war included burning and tingling of the feet, headache, insomnia, fatigue, and mental disturbances. The burning feet syndrome is most characteristic of deficiency, and animal studies suggest it is due to deterioration of the myelin sheath that coats and protects the nerves.

RISK FOR DEFICIENCY: There is little risk of deficiency, given that pantothenic acid is widely available in food. Deficiency can occur in severely malnourished individuals.

RDA/AI: Men: 5 mg Women: 5 mg
Pregnancy: 6 mg
Breastfeeding: 7 mg

DV: 10 mg

UL: Not determined. No harm has been seen with doses up to 1,200 mg/day. Much higher doses are known to cause GI upset.

SUPPLEMENT CONSIDERATIONS: For most individuals, a supplement providing 100 percent of the DV is adequate, though the 50 to 100 mg often found in "stress" B-vitamins is certainly safe. Most dietary supplements provide pantothenic acid as D-calcium pantothenate, though you might also see it as panto-thenol or pantethine. Some people supplement with royal jelly, a substance secreted by bees to feed their larvae, which naturally contains large amounts of pantothenic acid.

PARTNER NUTRIENTS: It is best to take pantothenic acid together with the others in the B-vitamin family.

SPECIAL POPULATIONS: None.

VITAMIN B6 (PYRIDOXINE)

Vitamin B6 is actually a group of compounds with similar activity. There are three primary forms of the vitamin: pyridoxine, which is primarily found in plants, and pyridoxal and pyridoxamine, which are most abundant in humans and animals. Vitamin B6 plays an important role in the production of fuel and energy, and is critical for optimal function of our brain and our nervous and immune systems. In spite of how important vitamin B6 is to our health, research shows that more than 30 million Americans are deficient in this important vitamin.

Most of the vitamin B6 we ingest travels to the liver, where it is converted to pyridoxal 5'-phosphate (PLP), the most biolog-ically active form. PLP then travels via the bloodstream to cells throughout the body. What is not readily used is stored in our muscles. PLP is what is measured in the blood to determine your vitamin B6 status.

WHAT IT DOES: Vitamin B6 is involved in many important bodily processes. It is vital for the metabolism of protein and the production of the heme found in hemoglobin. Indeed, a deficiency of vitamin B6 can lead to anemia characterized by small red blood cells and low levels of hemoglobin. B6, along with niacin, zinc, and magnesium, are necessary for the conversion of plant omega-3 (alpha-linolenic acid) to the long-chain omega-3 fatty acid DHA (docosahexaenoic acid), which is crucial for brain, eye, and cardiovascular health throughout our lives. Vitamin B6 is also needed to convert tryptophan to niacin.

Vitamin B6 is necessary for the brain to develop and function properly, and for the health of the protective myelin coating that surrounds our nerves. It is also involved in the production of the neurotransmitters gamma-aminobutyric acid (GABA), serotonin, norepinephrine, and dopamine, all of which positively affect mood. Low levels of B6 increase the risk for depression and impair cognition, attention, and memory.

Numerous studies have evaluated the use of vitamin B6 for treating the symptoms associated with premenstrual syndrome (PMS). A 2009 systematic review of clinical trials published in the *Canadian Journal of Pharmacology* concluded that vitamin B6 improves depression, anxiety, and breast tenderness associated with PMS. It's thought that B6 eases these symptoms via its effect on neurotransmitter production.

B6 is also effective for treating morning sickness in pregnancy. The American College of Obstetrics and Gynecology recommends that pregnant women who are experiencing nausea and vomiting take 10 to 25 mg of vitamin B6 every eight hours as first-line therapy for symptom alleviation.

Vitamin B6 is important for the manufacture of melatonin, a hormone that regulates our internal clock, allowing us to fall asleep naturally when nighttime falls. A deficiency in B6 can make it harder to fall and stay asleep. Melatonin also has potent antioxidant activity, supports the immune system, and plays a role in the regulation of female reproductive hormones. (For more on melatonin, see pages XXX–XXX.)

These days medical experts recognize that inflammation is driving many of the chronic diseases seen in Western countries—and it appears that vitamin B6 is part of this story. The Framingham Heart Study, a long-term investigation into the causes of heart disease, yielded so much important information that it was extended by enrolling the offspring of those in the original study. It was in this cohort that researchers made an interesting discovery. When scientists compared vitamin B6 levels and the levels of chemicals responsible for inflammation in 2,229 adults enrolled in the Framingham Offspring Study, they found that those with the highest levels of inflammation had the lowest levels of vitamin B6, as measured by blood levels of PLP. Studies also show that more than 50 percent of people with type-2 diabetes, a condition associated with inflammation and increased risk of cardiovascular disease, have low levels of PLP. Low PLP levels are also seen in those with rheumatoid arthritis and inflammatory bowel disease. In 2012, Tuft University researchers confirmed that as inflammation in the body rises, vitamin B6 levels fall, and that even marginally low PLP levels (20–30 nmol/L) are associated with an increased risk of coronary artery disease and stroke. Pretty scary when you really stop and think about it.

Vitamin B6, along with folic acid and vitamin B12, lowers elevated homocysteine levels. High levels of homocysteine have been associated with atherosclerosis, blood clots, heart attacks, and strokes. This same trio of B-vitamins was also shown in a large-scale study to reduce the risk of developing age-related macular degeneration.

And there is evidence that having adequate vitamin B6 on board may help protect us against cancer. A meta-analysis of 13 prospective studies published in 2010 in the *Journal of the American Medical Association* noted that B6 intake and PLP were inversely correlated with colorectal cancer risk, and that for every 0.1 nmol/L increase in serum PLP concentration, colorectal cancer risk decreased by 49 percent.

And last but not least: Calcium citrate and vitamin B6 are two supplements to consider if you've been plagued by calcium oxalate kidney stones, one of the most common types, as these nutrients help prevent oxalate from being absorbed.

FOOD SOURCES: The best sources of highly bioavailable vitamin B6 include tuna, salmon, turkey, beef, and chicken. Many plants contain B6 in the form of pyridoxine glucoside, which is less bioavailable but more stable when heated than the B6 in meat sources. Baked potatoes and sweet potatoes are very good sources of B6, as are avocados and bananas. Other sources include spinach, raw or fermented cruciferous vegetables (cauliflower, broccoli, cabbage), bell peppers, carrots, cooked soybeans, raisins, and canned green beans. It is very important to note than there is no requirement for fortification of grains with vitamin B6 even though there is for vitamins B1, B2, B3, folic acid, and iron.

SIGNS OF DEFICIENCY: Low levels of B6 can cause anemia from low heme production, as well as glossitis (red swollen tongue), gingivitis, burning mouth syndrome, cracking skin at the corners of the mouth, tingling and numbness in the feet and hands, fatigue, weakness, insomnia, depression, irritability, cognitive issues, dizziness, and seizures. Chronic deficiency may also increase the risk for kidney stones.

RISK FOR DEFICIENCY: The CDC Second National Report on Biochemical Indicators of Diet and Nutrition in the U.S. estimates that more than 30 million Americans are deficient in vitamin B6, of which 10 million are over the age of 40. Women are almost twice as likely to be deficient as men, and deficiency rates for blacks (15.7 percent) were higher than for whites (10.7 percent). Women may be at greater risk for deficiency because of their use of oral contraceptives and hormone therapy during menopause. (Estrogen lowers vitamin B6 levels.) I believe that since marginal vitamin B6 deficiency (PLP levels 20–30 nmol/L) have been associated with an increased risk for heart disease and other orders, the cutoff level of less than 20 nmol/L for deficiency underestimates the number of people with low vitamin B6 in the U.S. population.

Many of us are at risk for marginal vitamin B6 deficiency, given the growing number of inflammatory conditions we see in Western nations (obesity, diabetes, cardiovascular disease, diabetes, rheumatoid arthritis, autoimmune disorders, etc.). Vegetarians/vegans and those with kidney disease, liver disease, and absorption problems (such as from Crohn's disease, ulcerative colitis, and celiac disease) may also be at risk for B6 deficiency. Alcoholics and heavy drinkers are very likely to be deficient in B6 as well as thiamine, riboflavin, and other B-vitamins. Pregnant and breastfeeding women have increased needs for vitamin B6.

RDA/AI: Men, before age 50: mg   Women, before age 50:
1.3 mg   1.3 mg
After 50: 1.7 mg after 50   After 50: 1.5 mg
Pregnancy: 1.9 mg
Breastfeeding 2. 0 mg

DV: 20 mg

UL: 100 mg

SUPPLEMENT CONSIDERATIONS: In supplements, B6 can appear be listed as pyridoxal, pyridoxamine, pyridoxine hydrochloride, or pyridoxal 5'-phosphate (P5P or PLP). I generally recommend 20 to 30 mg per day as P5P or PLP, which provides significantly more than the RDA and is probably much closer to the amount we actually need.

PARTNER NUTRIENTS: Riboflavin is needed to convert all forms of vitamin B6 to the bioactive PLP in the liver. Then, cells need zinc to take up and use the PLP. A deficiency in zinc or riboflavin will contribute to vitamin B6 deficiency. And your body requires B6 to convert tryptophan to niacin, which is just one more reason to take your B-vitamins together!

SPECIAL POPULATIONS: Pregnant and breastfeeding women have a greater need for vitamin B6, as is noted by the higher RDA. Unfortunately, small red blood cells and low hemoglobin can indicate either iron deficiency anemia or the anemia caused by low B6. Since iron *and* vitamin B6 levels start dropping after the second trimester, it is important for a woman to make sure she is getting adequate amounts of both! To make sure the baby is getting plenty of vitamin B6, breastfeeding mothers should continue taking their prenatal vitamin. Researchers have found that it takes double the RDA of vitamin B6, or more, to maintain adequate levels in breast milk.

BIOTIN (VITAMIN B7)

Biotin is a water-soluble vitamin necessary for the metabolism of carbohydrates, fats, and the amino acids found in protein. If you've ever strolled the supplement aisles in search of a vitamin that might improve the health of your hair, skin, or nails, you've likely come across biotin. It is used to treat hoof problems in horses, which led investigators to study its use in human nails. Several small studies suggest biotin can improve thin, brittle nails when taken at doses of 2.5 mg per day for at least six months. Unfortunately, there is virtually no evidence that biotin can help improve thinning hair, a condition for which it is commonly promoted.

WHAT IT DOES: Biotin is necessary for the synthesis of fatty acids and for making glucose from sources other than carbohydrates. There may be a relationship between biotin levels in the body and blood sugar, as some studies suggest that biotin supplements, alone or in combination with chromium, might improve blood sugar and triglycerides in people with type 1 and type 2 diabetes.

Biotin is also involved in the production of an enzyme that makes the protective myelin sheath that surrounds our nerves. A small pilot study published in 2015 in the journal *Multiple Sclerosis and Related Disorders* found that high doses of biotin (100–600 mg per day) slowed the progression of multiple sclerosis (MS) in 21 of 23 patients. Two randomized placebo controlled trials are currently under way to see if indeed biotin might be beneficial for those living with MS.

We are also learning that many women develop a marginal biotin deficiency during pregnancy, which is concerning given that animal studies show that maternal biotin deficiency can cause cleft lip and cleft palate in the animal's offspring. It appears that biotin, like folic acid, is a vital nutrient for developing embryos. The good news is that a basic supplement can readily restore levels, as was seen in a 2002 study published in the *American Journal of Clinical Nutrition* that showed that healthy pregnant women with marginal biotin deficiency saw their levels return to normal after taking 300 *mcg of* biotin (10 times the RDA) for 2 weeks.

FOOD SOURCES: Biotin is present naturally in a wide variety of foods, with the highest amounts found in milk, meat, eggs, peanuts, almonds, oats, yeast, sweet potatoes, and cereals.

The bacteria that inhabit the GI tract can also synthesize small amounts of biotin.

SIGNS OF DEFICIENCY: Hair loss and/or thinning of the hair, cracking at the corners of the mouth, dry eyes, and a scaly red rash around the eyes, nose, mouth, or genital area can all indicate low levels of biotin. With more severe deficiency, depression, fatigue, hallucinations, and tingling in the arms and legs can occur.

RISK FOR DEFICIENCY: Multiple studies suggest that many women become marginally biotin deficient during pregnancy. Smoking increases the metabolism of biotin, which could lead to deficiency. Raw egg whites contain avidin, an antimicrobial protein that binds biotin and prevents it from being absorbed. Biotin deficiency can be induced in as little as three weeks in experimental studies where people eat raw egg whites two to three times per day. This is not an issue for the vast majority of us, however, as avidin is destroyed when eggs are cooked. And finally, some babies are born with biotinidase deficiency, a genetic defect that prevents the body from being able to utilize biotin. It requires lifelong supplementation.

RDA/AI: Men: 30 mcg   Women: 30 mcg
                          Pregnancy: 30 mcg
                          Breastfeeding: 35 mcg

DV: 300 mcg (roughly 10 times higher than the RDA)

UL: None established. Studies in healthy individuals failed to show any adverse effects when taking 5 mg per day for two years. Studies using doses of up to 300 mg per day have not shown any significant adverse effects other than diarrhea.

SUPPLEMENT CONSIDERATIONS: A multivitamin or B-complex supplement that provides the 300 mcg per day of biotin is sufficient for most people. If you have brittle nails, taking 2.5 mg per day for a few months is a reasonable approach. If you have multiple sclerosis, talk to your health-care provider to see if a high dose of biotin might be an option for you.

PARTNER NUTRIENTS: B-vitamins are best taken together either in a multivitamin or B-complex supplement. Biotin and chromium taken together may improve blood sugar control in diabetics.

SPECIAL POPULATIONS: There's growing evidence that pregnancy increases the metabolism of biotin and that women may develop a marginal biotin deficiency during the latter half of pregnancy. Biotin is necessary for the baby's normal growth; animal studies indicate low biotin levels may cause birth defects. A prenatal vitamin containing 150 to 300 mcg per day of biotin should be taken throughout pregnancy and while nursing.

FOLATE (VITAMIN B9)

Armed with a medical degree from the London School of Medicine for Women, Lucy Wills, an English physician born in 1898, traveled to Bombay, India, to study a particular type of anemia common there among poor pregnant women. The type of anemia she observed, megaloblastic macrocytic anemia, is marked by large, immature red blood cells with a short life span. This anemia is different from that seen with iron deficiency, in which there are small red blood cells with low levels of hemoglobin (microcytic hypochromic anemia). Dr. Wills surmised that a nutritional deficiency was involved and found that giving women brewer's yeast, or a yeast extract called Marmite, could readily prevent the anemia. However, it wasn't until the early 1940s that researchers identified folate as the substance in yeast responsible for this effect. (Vitamin B12 deficiency can also cause megaloblastic macrocytic anemia.)

Decades later, doctors found that higher blood folate levels decreased the risk of a specific category of birth defects: neural tube defects (NTD), such as spina bifida and anencephaly, which are caused by the incomplete closing of the spine and skull. In September 1992, the U.S. Public Health Service recommended that to reduce the risk of NTD, all women who could become pregnant get 400 mcg per day of folic acid, the synthetic form of folate. In 1998, the FDA required the fortification of cereals and flour products with folic acid. Today, the U.S. Preventive Task Force recommends that all women planning or capable of pregnancy take a daily supplement containing 400 to 800 mcg of folic acid.

Vitamin B9 comes in two primary forms: Folate occurs naturally in food, whereas folic acid, which is synthetic, is used in dietary supplements and in food fortification. Folate is derived from the Latin word for leaf, *folium,* because it was first identified in spinach and green leafy vegetables. The term *folate* refers to both the naturally occurring folate and folic acid.

WHAT IT DOES: Folate is vital for growth and development and for maintaining healthy brain function, protecting us from certain cancers, and preventing a rise in homocysteine. High blood levels of homocysteine (a condition known as hyperhomocysteinemia) have been associated with an increased risk of heart disease, stroke, and peripheral vascular disease. As we started with folate's importance in pregnancy, let's start there and dive a little deeper.

In the womb, the baby's cells are dividing at an extraordinary rate to allow for the rapid growth. Folate is needed to make new DNA during cell division. Without adequate folic acid, DNA synthesis and cell division are hindered, increasing the risk for miscarriage and NTD. Folate fortification of cereal and grain products, as well as increased public awareness due to the efforts of the government and the March of Dimes, has led to a decline of NTD in the U.S. However, annually there are still roughly 3,000 cases of spina bifida or anencephaly, an absence of a major portion of the brain, skull, and scalp. The end of the neural tube that becomes the baby's head closes 23 to 26 *days* after conception, which is why physicians recommend that folic acid be started at least one month before a woman gets pregnant, to ensure adequate levels. According to CDC data, Latinas have lower blood folate levels, are less likely to consume foods fortified with folic acid, and have the highest rate of NTD when compared to black or white women.

Remember Dr. Wills and her investigation of the anemia in poor women living in India? Folate is involved in making red blood cells. When folate levels are low, red blood cell precursors, called megaloblasts, are unable to fully mature—and many are destroyed in the bone marrow by white blood cells. Those megaloblasts that survive appear large, but the inner contents of their cells are not completely developed, leading them to die prematurely and leaving the body depleted of essential red blood cells.

Folate and vitamins B6 and B12 are important regulators of the metabolism of homocysteine, an amino acid in our blood. When blood levels of these B-vitamins are low, homocysteine rises, increasing the risk of stroke and heart disease. Although this relationship has been well established, studies using folate and/or other B-vitamins have not shown consistent protection against heart attacks or improvement in atherosclerosis. Despite this, the American Heart Association has said that those with elevated homocysteine, who at high risk for heart disease and stroke, "should be strongly advised to be sure to get enough folic acid and vitamins B6 and B-12 in their diet." *Bottom line: Taking a daily multivitamin will help ensure that you are getting adequate levels of vitamins B6, B9, and B12.*

A large-scale study reported in the *Journal of the American Medical Association* in March 2015 helps to support the recommendation of the American Heart Association. Strokes are the second leading cause of death in the world and the number one cause of death in China, where the China Stroke Primary Prevention Trial was conducted. The study included more than 20,000 adults in China with high blood pressure but no history of stroke or heart attack. These patients were randomly prescribed a single pill containing 10 mg of enalapril (a medication used to treat hypertension) alone, or 10 mg of enalapril plus 800 mcg of folic acid. The average duration of treatment was four and one half years. Astonishingly, the combination pill significantly reduced the risk of having a stroke compared to the enalapril alone. Researchers found that those with the lowest baseline plasma folate levels had the greatest protection against stroke. However, it is important to note that China does not fortify its grains with folate, so the benefits for the study participants might have been greater than what we would see in countries with fortification programs in place.

One area that is relatively new in the medical scene is the realization that not everyone has the right genetic machinery to metabolize and activate certain nutrients. This appears to be particularly true when it comes to converting supplemental folic acid to its active form, L-methylfolate. Because most studies used folic acid, and a significant number of people may not have been able to fully convert it, this could explain some of the negative findings. *Bottom line: There are genetic tests available to determine if one has this mutation, called the MTHFR genetic mutation. However, since it is unclear when and who to test, it makes sense to choose a supplement that contains the active form of folic acid.*

Low folate and high homocysteine levels may contribute to the deterioration in cognitive and mental function in elders. A study by researchers at Oxford University published in 2013 in the *Proceedings of the National Academy of Sciences*, found that two years of high-dose B-vitamin treatment (folic acid 800 mcg, vitamin B6 20 mg, vitamin B12 500 mcg) slowed the shrinkage of whole brain volume in elder individuals with an increased risk of dementia. Using MRI imaging, this study also found that the B-vitamins reduced atrophy in regions of the brain specifically vulnerable to Alzheimer's disease—by as much as sevenfold! This is consistent with a large study in the Netherlands that found that when men and women (50–70 years old) with high homocysteine levels took 800 mcg per day of folic acid for three years, it increased memory and other measures of cognitive function. It's important to point out that this benefit is probably only seen in those with low blood levels of folate. *Bottom line: If you or someone you love is having loss of memory or early signs of dementia, make sure folate, B6, and B12 levels are checked! If they are low, work with your health-care provider to ensure that they are corrected.*

Folate plays a role in the production of neurotransmitters, including serotonin. This may explain why folate deficiency has been associated with depressed mood and a poorer response to antidepressant medications. Some studies have found that supplementing antidepressant therapy with folic acid can improve treatment, but there's no evidence that folate alone can treat depression.

FOOD SOURCES: Other than beef liver, which contains the highest amount of folate, the plant kingdom offers the best sources for meeting your daily requirement of this vital nutrient. The dark green leafy vegetables, lettuce, kale, and cooked spinach, as well as other green vegetables, such as asparagus, broccoli, and Brussels sprouts, are excellent sources. Folate is also found in avocados, oranges, papayas, bananas, tomato juice, nuts and seeds, legumes, and fortified grains and cereals.

SIGNS OF DEFICIENCY: Folate deficiency can cause megaloblastic anemia, leading to poor concentration, headaches, irritability, fatigue, and shortness of breath. Symptoms of deficiency also include gastrointestinal upset, particularly abdominal pain and diarrhea after eating; sore beefy red, shiny tongue, and darkening of the skin in the creases of the palms and soles. Low levels can cause an elevation of the amino acid homocysteine, which is associated with an increased risk of heart disease, stroke, peripheral vascular disease, and cognitive decline in elders.

RISK FOR DEFICIENCY: Heavy drinkers, people with absorption problems such as Crohn's or celiac disease; those with genetic abnormalities that prevent activation of folate, zinc deficiency, low stomach acid, and/or small bowel intestinal overgrowth (SIBO) are all at risk for deficiency. The CDC Second National Report on Biochemical Indicators of Diet and Nutrition in the U.S. found that non-Hispanic blacks had the lowest folate levels when compared to Hispanics and non-Hispanic whites, and more than 15 million Americans over the age of 20 have elevated homocysteine (>13 µmol/L), which could be due to either low folate or vitamin B12.

RDA/AI: Men: 400 mcg

Women: 400 mcg
Pregnancy: 600 mcg
Breastfeeding: 500 mcg

DV: 400 mcg

UL: 1,000 mcg

SUPPLEMENT CONSIDERATIONS: When grains are processed, their nutrient rich outer covering and inner germ layer are removed, taking with them most of the valuable vitamins and minerals. By law, companies must add back the B-vitamins that are lost in the process, including folate. Because the U.S. fortifies cereals and grains with folic acid, making recommendations for how much folic acid should take in a supplement is really difficult. Some of us actually consume very little processed grain, preferring 100 percent whole-grain pasta and breads, which often are not fortified. But many people consume only fortified cereals and grains and could easily reach the upper limit of 1,000 mcg per day of folate from their food and taking supplements.

The reason we are concerned about not getting too much folic acid is because there have been some data linking folic acid supplements and folic acid food fortification with an increased risk of cancer. A 2013 systematic review by the *U.S. Preventive Services Task Force* failed to find any association between folic acid supplements and cancer however, other reviews have suggested a possible link with colorectal and prostate cancer.

So, who should supplement? Women who could become pregnant should supplement with 400 mcg per day of folic acid. Pregnant women should take 600 mcg per day. Those who are at risk for deficiency or who have early signs of dementia should have their blood folate levels checked and corrected if low. For the rest of us, I would recommend a multivitamin that provides 200 mcg (if you regularly eat processed foods or breakfast cereal) or 400 mcg (if you eat a diet low in grains) of the active form of folic acid, usually listed on the label as L-methylfolate or 5-methyltetrahydrofolate (5-MTHF). I do not recommend taking higher doses of folic acid unless there is documented evidence of deficiency or upon the recommendation of a qualified health-care practitioner.

PARTNER NUTRIENTS: Vitamins B6, B12, and folate should be taken together, even if you need to take a higher amount in a separate supplement of any particular one. Zinc is necessary for the absorption of folate, and vitamin C assists in the conversion of folate to its active form.

SPECIAL POPULATIONS: Women who could become pregnant, or who are pregnant, should ensure that they are getting adequate amounts of folate.

VITAMIN B12 (COBALAMIN)

In the mid-19th century, English physician Thomas Addison described a lethal form of anemia in which the skin and lips grew pale, the tongue became red and shiny, the gait became abnormal, the hands and feet tingled, and even the smallest amount of exertion left the individual breathless. He hypothesized that it might have something to do with a disease of the stomach. In 1872, this cluster of symptoms was given the name *pernicious anemia* by the German physician Anton Biermer. *Pernicious* is derived from the Latin *perniciosus,* which means "destructive," as all cases of pernicious anemia at the time were fatal.

During the early 20th century, a physician named George Whipple discovered that feeding liver to anemic dogs effectively resolved the condition. Intrigued by Whipple's work, two other physicians, George Minot and William Murphy reported that they had cured 45 human patients with pernicious anemia by feeding them large quantities of raw liver. The effects were dramatic and quick, with symptoms resolving within two weeks. For this amazing breakthrough, Drs. Minot, Murphy, and Whipple shared the Nobel Prize for Physiology or Medicine in 1934.

William Castle, a physician at Harvard, found that when people had their stomach removed, they still died of pernicious anemia even when given copious amounts of raw liver. He postulated that there must be something "intrinsic" in the stomach that was necessary to absorb the particular nutrient in liver that could cure the disease.

Vitamin B12 was eventually identified in 1948, fully characterized in 1956 and finally synthesized in 1971. And Dr. Castle was correct. Parietal cells in the stomach secrete a substance, gastric intrinsic factor, which is necessary for the absorption of vitamin B12 in the small intestine. Vitamin B12, amongst its many roles, is necessary for the production of healthy red blood cells and prolonged deficiency, as in pernicious anemia, leaves the body without enough red blood cells to carry oxygen to all our tissues. If not corrected, this lack of red blood cells damages the heart, nerves, brain, and other organs, eventually leading to death. It took the work of many dedicated physicians and researchers to unlock the powerful role B12 plays in our health.

Vitamin B12 is a water-soluble nutrient that is essential for the maintenance of blood and nerve cells and the formation of DNA in all our cells. Vitamin B12 is naturally present in meat and seafood; it is added to fortify cereals and is available in dietary supplements and as a prescription drug. Of the 13 essential vitamins, it is the only one that contains the trace mineral cobalt, which is why vitamin B12 is also referred to as cobalamin.

WHAT IT DOES: Vitamin B12 is a real power player when it comes to maintaining the health of our brain and cells. We need it for physical and mental energy, as well as emotional well-being. Vitamin B12 contributes to the production of myelin, the protective covering of our nerves, which explains why a deficiency causes tingling and burning in our arms and legs.

Vitamin B12, along with B6 and folate, plays an important role in the production of the neurotransmitters serotonin, dopamine, and norepinephrine, chemicals in the brain that are responsible for mood and pleasure. Low levels of vitamin B12 can lead to depression, confusion, and possibly even dementia. In patients with low vitamin B12 levels, the improvement I've witnessed in their mood and energy has often been dramatic once their levels were back in the normal range.

Just like folate, vitamin B12 is needed during pregnancy to ensure the healthy development of the baby. The requirements for vitamin B12 are increased during pregnancy and even marginally low levels may increase a woman's risk for postpartum depression. Anyone who is suffering from depression should have basic laboratory testing done to ensure that a nutritional deficiency is not part of the problem.

In concert with other B-vitamins, namely B6 and folate, vitamin B12 is important for creating and maintaining our DNA and for helping the liver do its job of detoxification. Just as with folate, if you don't have enough B12, the amino acid homocysteine builds up in the body. Elevated homocysteine causes estrogens to accumulate, which may be why some researchers believe B12 (and possibly folate) may help protect women against breast cancer. Because B12 is important for the functioning of our red and white blood cells, deficiency can cause megaloblastic anemia and a diminished immune response. (See *megaloblastic anemia* under "folate," on page XXX).

Many of us are concerned about preserving our memory and keeping our mind sharp throughout our lives. A scientific review of more than 40 studies found that low levels of vitamin B12 are associated with dementia, Alzheimer's, and Parkinson's disease. I want to stress that these conditions have multifactorial causes and that there are many pieces to the puzzle, but one part of a holistic prevention strategy would be to make sure we are getting enough vitamin B12. The American Academy of Neurology recommends that elders in general, and anyone with suspected dementia in particular, be checked for B12 deficiency.

And if all this wasn't enough, there's also some evidence that vitamin B12 taken alongside its famous sidekicks folic acid and vitamin B6 may help prevent macular degeneration—and 1,000 mcg/d of sublingually administered vitamin B12 alone may be beneficial for those with recurrent mouth ulcers.

Given how very important vitamin B12 is for our health, it might surprise you to know that many of us may have lower than optimal levels. Vitamin B12 is found almost exclusively in animal foods and requires three steps for absorption. Once the food enters the stomach, hydrochloric acid and the digestive enzyme pepsin act upon the food to separate the B12 from the protein that it is attached to. This free vitamin B12 is then joined to a protein called gastric intrinsic factor (IF), made by the parietal cells in the stomach. The B12-IF then travels to the very end of the small intestine where, if calcium supplies are adequate, it is absorbed.

Can you see where problems might arise? As vitamin B12 is found in animal foods (meat, seafood, dairy), vegans and vegetarian are at risk for deficiency. No matter what might read, you cannot get vitamin B12 by eating nonfortified grains, nutritional yeast, algae, or seaweed. If you suddenly stop consuming all animal products, you'll be fine for a few years because you can use the vitamin B12 stored in your liver. However, babies born to vegans and then exclusively breastfed are at high risk for B12 deficiency because they have no reserve in their liver. Just one more reason women should take a prenatal vitamin during pregnancy and while breastfeeding.

The second part of the journey involves stomach acid. You can absorb vitamin B12 without stomach acid if it isn't attached to protein—such as in a vitamin or in fortified breakfast cereal. But you can't separate vitamin B12 from animal protein without it. As we get older, we make less stomach acid. In fact, up to 30 percent of people over the age of 50 are at risk for vitamin B12 deficiency, which is why the Institute of Medicine recommends that people aged 50 and older take supplemental vitamin B12, either as a vitamin and/or by increasing their intake of fortified cereals.

One of the primary reasons many people have insufficient stomach acid, however, is the widespread use of PPIs (Nexium, Prilosec, Prevacid) and H2 blockers (Tagamet, Pepcid), whose job is to shut off the acid-producing pumps in the stomach. More than 118 million prescriptions were written for PPIs in the United States in 2010, which doesn't include all the over-the-counter purchases of PPIs and H2 blockers. The long-term use of these drugs may be a double whammy. When taking these medications, you can't separate the vitamin B12 from the protein in your food because you don't have enough stomach acid. There is also some question whether these drugs also impair calcium absorption. (The FDA mandates a warning on all PPIs that they increase the risk of fracture.) Short-term use of these drugs (2–6 months) is not likely to cause problems, but many people take them for years. Eventually, you are likely to develop a B12 deficiency.

Even setting aside the question of calcium absorption and PPIs, B12 deficiency alone may be bad for your bones. The Framingham Osteoporosis Study showed a relationship between B12 deficiency and osteoporosis in both men and women. Other researchers have found that the higher the level of homocysteine, which indicates a deficiency in vitamins B6, B9 and/or B12, the greater the risk of fracture. Because B12 is important to DNA synthesis, a deficiency likely leads to lower levels of bone-forming cells, resulting in weakened bones that are more likely to break.

And there's a third essential step in B12's journey through your digestive system. Assuming you ate your chicken and there was sufficient stomach acid to separate the protein and the B12, you still need intrinsic factor (IF) to grab hold of that free B12 and carry it down to the small intestine where it can be absorbed. Some people are unable to make IF and develop pernicious anemia, the anemia of B12 deficiency identified nearly 200 years ago. Pernicious anemia can develop as you age (it is most commonly diagnosed after the age of 60) when the lining of the stomach weakens and destroys the parietal cells that make IF (a condition called atrophic gastritis). An infection with *Helicobacter pylori,* a bacterium that can cause ulcers, can also damage the parietal cells. Pernicious anemia can result secondary to an autoimmune disorder where your own immune system attacks the IF protein or the cells responsible for making it. Those with a history of Graves' disease or other autoimmune disorders should be closely monitored as they may increase the risk of pernicious anemia, which requires lifelong B12 supplementation.

The final stage of our journey is absorption across the intestinal tract. You need both IF and calcium to absorb B12. Sometimes, people may have had this part of their small intestine, the ileum, removed due to disease, making it impossible to absorb vitamin B12 when it's taken orally. In these cases, B12 injections or nasal spray are usually necessary.

While we are unsure of the exact mechanism, the popular diabetes drug metformin (Glucophage) depletes vitamin B12. Studies show that people who have been on metformin for more than four years have an increased risk of B12 deficiency. I am sure that early in my medical career I missed this in some of my diabetic patients. The numbness and tingling, or neuropathy in their feet, is a common complication of advanced diabetes, and so we simply added another drug to relieve the symptoms. I am far more diligent and far more aware of the impact of nutritional deficiencies on my patients' health these days. *Bottom line: If you have diabetes and are taking metformin, your health-care provider should check your B12 level annually.*

FOOD SOURCES: Beef, clams, seafood, poultry, eggs, and dairy products are the best natural sources of vitamin B12. Some cereal grains are fortified with vitamin B12.

SIGNS OF DEFICIENCY: No single sign has been uniquely associated with inadequate levels of vitamin B12. And by the time signs and symptoms are present, deficiency has often been present for some time. Symptoms can include pale skin, fatigue, dizziness, sore tongue, shortness of breath, and heart palpitations, along with neurological changes including tingling in the hands and feet, weakness, depression, paranoia, and personality changes. It's important to catch B12 deficiency early, because some neurological effects are irreversible.

RISK FOR DEFICIENCY: In the CDC Second National Report on Biochemical Indicators of Diet and Nutrition in the U.S. Population, more than 18 million people have B12 deficiency. Non-Hispanic whites had the highest incidence of deficiency. Two-thirds of those who are deficient are over the age of 40, with people over 60 being at greatest risk. That's because the risk of developing vitamin B12 deficiency increases with age due to decreased production of stomach acid and/or increased risk of pernicious anemia—and possibly due to medication use. People who have had gastric surgery (removal of the ileum or stomach) or bariatric surgery for weight loss are also at high risk for B12 deficiency. Vegans should take a B12 supplement and/or eat fortified cereal products.

RDA/AI: Men: 2.4 mcg   Women: 2.4 mcg

Pregnant: 2.6 mcg

Breastfeeding: 2.8 mcg

DV: 6 mcg

UL: The Food and Nutrition Board has not established a UL for vitamin B12 because of its low potential for toxicity. Large doses (1,000 mcg or higher) may cause diarrhea and itching in some people.

SUPPLEMENT CONSIDERATIONS: Cyanocobalamin is a synthetic form of vitamin B12 used in many dietary supplements and to fortify cereal grains. I recommend purchasing a supplement that contains methylcobalamin, the form your body wants and needs.

How much do you need? More than the RDA, that's for sure. I recommend you look for a supplement that provides four times the DV—roughly 25 mcg, particularly if you are over the age of 50. If you are taking medications that deplete B12 or have a medical condition that impairs absorption, make sure you get your vitamin B12 level checked. For most people, oral vitamin B12 is as effective as B12 shots for treating a deficiency, provided that a large enough oral dose is used (500–1,000 mcg per day).

WARNING!
People with Leber's Disease Should Avoid B12 Supplements

Leber's disease is a rare hereditary eye disease. Do not take vitamin B12 if you have this disease as it can harm the optic nerve, which might lead to blindness.

PARTNER NUTRIENTS: Folate and vitamins B6 and B12 are partners that work together to maintain our health. Large doses of folic acid can mask a vitamin B12 deficiency, which can be very dangerous as the nerve damage caused by B12 deficiency is often irreversible. Take your B-vitamins together, which is how they are found in multivitamins and B-complex supplements. Low levels of calcium can impair absorption of B12, so make sure you are getting enough in your diet.

SPECIAL POPULATIONS: Low vitamin B12 levels during pregnancy may increase the risk for neural tube defects (NTD). Exclusively breastfed infants of vegan mothers are at risk for vitamin B12 deficiency, which can have serious adverse consequences. Those over the age of 50 should take 25 to 50 mcg of supplemental vitamin B12.

VITAMIN C

Scurvy, a disease that results from a prolonged lack of vitamin C, was known in ancient times. Hippocrates described the symptoms of bleeding gums, easy bruising, poorly healing wounds, fatigue, depression, seizures, and death. Scurvy was common when sailors were out to sea for long stretches of time and subsisted primarily on meat and grain. While early explorers and physicians postulated that fresh foods could prevent scurvy, it wasn't until 1747 that the Scottish naval surgeon James Lind proved that citrus fruits could both prevent and treat the disease. Even with this knowledge, however, scurvy continued to plague sailors and soldiers all the way up through World War I.

Sailors weren't the only ones to develop scurvy. It was common during the great potato famine in Ireland. Scurvy suddenly appeared in infants during the latter part of the 19th and early 20th centuries, as women began to bottle feed their babies using heated milk, which destroys vitamin C. Physicians recommended that bottle-fed babies also be fed fruit juices to prevent the disease.

It wasn't until the 1930s that Albert Szent-Györgyi finally identified and isolated vitamin C. Vitamin C, or ascorbic acid, is a water-soluble vitamin that is made by most animals but must be consumed regularly in the diet of humans. Studies have shown that it takes remarkably little vitamin C, only 10 mg per day, to prevent scurvy. While we may not be seeing scurvy, roughly 16 million people in the U.S. are deficient in vitamin C.

WHAT IT DOES: Vitamin C has many duties to perform in the body. It is involved in maintaining a healthy immune response, which is why so many people reach for the vitamin C when they feel a cold coming on. Vitamin C enhances the activity of T-cells, macrophages, and other immune cells, helping to fight off infections and reduce the severity of allergic reactions. In 2013, the Cochrane Group, a prestigious organization that includes researchers and health-care professionals from around the world and offers high-quality health information, reviewed the research on vitamin C and colds. It concluded that given its low cost and the numerous studies that show a reduction in colds, people who frequently get upper respiratory infections should decide for themselves if it is worthwhile taking extra supplemental C. I definitely bump up my levels when traveling to give myself an extra edge against colds, flus, and infections. I also recommend extra vitamin C to all of my asthma patients to protect against respiratory infection and reduce exercise-induced asthma attacks.

And vitamin C can help more than just colds. A double-blinded study published in the British medical journal *Lancet* reported that 1,500 mg of vitamin C worked as well as the antibiotic azithromycin for the treatment of acute bronchitis. We overprescribe antibiotics, and since they aren't necessary for the more than 90 percent of acute bronchitis cases that are caused by viruses, taking vitamin C (and zinc) for bronchitis makes sense.

Vitamin C levels decline rapidly during periods of illness and emotional and physical strain. This may be one more reason why people perceive that they get sick more often when they are under persistent stress. Vitamin C also plays a role in activating folic acid, assists in the conversion of tryptophan to serotonin, and is a cofactor in the synthesis of carnitine, thyroxin, norepinephrine, and dopamine. Serotonin, norepinephrine, and dopamine are critical for maintaining a healthy mood and feeling pleasure in our lives. Carnitine is an amino acid that is important for turning fat into energy. Without adequate amounts of vitamin C, carnitine cannot be used properly, partly explaining the severe fatigue that occurs in scurvy.

Vitamin C is a powerful antioxidant and studies show that the higher the dietary intake, the lower the risk of certain cancers. A 2014 meta-analysis of studies in *PLoS One* (a journal of the Public Library of Science) found that just 100 mg per day of vitamin C reduced gastric cancer by 26 percent. A 2014 meta-analysis published in the *European Journal of Cancer* that included 17,696 breast cancer cases found that those who took vitamin C supplementation after their diagnoses reduced their risk of dying from cancer by 19 percent. Other studies have found that a high intake of dietary vitamin C is associated with a lower risk of esophageal, mouth, pancreatic, cervical, and rectal cancer. Vitamin C is just one of a number of critical nutrients in fruits and vegetables that help our body defend itself from cancer. Eat up!

Vitamin C is necessary for the synthesis of collagen, a structural protein found in skin and connective tissue. There it plays an important role in the healing of wounds and maintaining the health of our gums. As vitamin C levels fall and our ability to synthesize collagen becomes impaired, we begin to bruise more easily, our skin becomes thick and dry, wounds take longer to heal, and our joints begin to hurt. I recommend my patients take

300 to 500 mg of vitamin C twice a day for a few weeks before and after surgery to help support the healing process.

Gout is a painful condition in which uric acid crystallizes within the joints, often the big toe. The risk of gout increases with age, as well with obesity and diabetes, which increase uric acid levels in the body. Vitamin C helps reduce blood levels of uric acid. Studies show that 500 mg of vitamin C taken two times per day is beneficial for gout.

Vitamin C is an important nutrient during pregnancy. Low levels have been associated with an increased risk of preterm birth and premature rupture of membranes, which can be very dangerous to the mother and baby. Vitamin C may be particularly important for pregnant women who smoke. Researchers at the University of Alabama found that giving pregnant smokers vitamins C and E starting at 9 to 16 weeks' gestation significantly reduced the risk of placental abruption and preterm birth. Another study published in the *Journal of the American Medical Association* randomized 179 pregnant smokers to receive 500 mg per day of vitamin C or placebo throughout pregnancy and then followed their babies for an additional 12 months. The researchers found that maternal vitamin C improved the lung function of the newborns and decreased wheezing through the one-year follow-up. Clearly it is best to not smoke, especially during pregnancy, but taking extra vitamin C in conjunction with a prenatal vitamin can help reduce some of the risk to mom and baby.

Vitamin C is important for reproductive function in men. In Western nations, sperm counts have fallen by roughly 50 percent over the last 50 years and sperm quality has also declined. This may be due to increasing exposure to environmental chemicals and toxins including tobacco and heavy metals, resulting in increased oxidative stress in the testes, where sperm is produced. Seminal fluid is normally rich in vitamin C, where it acts as a potent antioxidant and helps to maintain the quality and function of sperm. Studies have found that fertile men have significantly higher seminal vitamin C levels compared to infertile men. Vitamin C at doses of 500 mg two times per day in combination with other antioxidants may help improve male fertility.

A little known fact is that taking vitamin C before having a procedure or scan using contrast material can help prevent acute kidney injury. A meta-analysis of nine randomized studies published in the *Journal of the American College of Cardiology* found that patients taking vitamin C before having coronary angiography had 33 percent less risk of contrast-induced acute kidney injury when compared with patients receiving placebo. I generally recommend taking 500 mg of vitamin C 1 to 2 hours before undergoing any elective scan with contrast (CT with contrast, etc.).

And finally, vitamin C is important for skin health. It helps wounds heal and topical preparations that contain 5 to 10 percent of ascorbic acid can reduce the appearance of wrinkles.

FOOD SOURCES: When you hear vitamin C, you probably think of citrus fruits but it is also found in high concentrations in peaches, peppers (sweet and chile), papayas, strawberries, broccoli, and other fruits and vegetables. Vitamin C is plentiful in sardines and organ meats; unfortunately, these are not part of the typical American diet. Remember, vitamin C levels fall during cooking and with prolonged storage.

SIGNS OF DEFICIENCY: Common signs of vitamin C deficiency include fatigue, swollen bleeding gums, easy bruising, thickened skin, dry hair, and poorly healing wounds. Because vitamin C is needed to enhance the absorption of non-heme (plant-based) iron, those who do not consume meat or fish may have a higher risk for iron deficiency.

RISK FOR DEFICIENCY: The CDC Second National Report on Biochemical Indicators of Diet and Nutrition in the U.S. Population found that almost 16 million people in the U.S. over the age of six are deficient in vitamin C, taking in less than 30 mg/day—far less than the 75 to 90 mg recommended by the RDA, which itself is far lower than most experts believe is optimal. The lowest concentrations were seen among 20- to 59-year-olds. The biggest risk for deficiency is lack of fresh fruit and vegetables in the diet. People with malabsorption disorders or kidney disease may also be at risk for deficiency. The need for vitamin C is increased due to illness, stress (emotional or physical), inflammatory disorders, low stomach acid, smoking, hyperthyroidism, iron deficiency, surgery, burns, and low intake of protein.

RDA/AI: Men: 90 mg   Women: 75 mg
Pregnancy: 85 mg
Breastfeeding: 20 mg
Smokers: RDA plus an additional 35 mg per day

DV: 60 mg

UL: 2,000 mg

SUPPLEMENT CONSIDERATIONS: Some people are really good about eating those 4 to 5 cups of fresh fruits and vegetables every single day, but most of us fall short. I definitely think that with all the pollution and environmental toxins we are exposed to, we need more than the DV, which is only 60 mg. It takes approximately 400 mg per day to saturate our tissues, so I generally recommend supplementing with 200 to 300 mg per day. Natural (rose hips or acerola) and synthetic forms of vitamin C will both get the job done, though nothing can come close to all the supportive phytonutrients you get when you actually eat an orange or bowl of berries.

Absorption decreases as you increase the dose: Almost one hundred percent of doses up to 200 mg are absorbed, compared to only 63 percent of a 500 mg dose. If you are feeling sick, taking 200 mg several times per day is better than taking 2,000 mg all at once. Vitamin C is water soluble, so it's hard to get too much and it is rapidly lost if not continually replaced in the diet. The main reason the UL has been set at 2,000 mg is because large doses cause loose stools and mild gastrointestinal distress. There are buffered forms of vitamin C that don't cause the gastrointestinal upset associated with plain ascorbic acid. After opening your vitamin C, store it in a closed container in a dark area, as exposure to air and light can reduce its potency.

Prolonged use of high-potency chewable vitamin C (500 mg) has been associated with erosion of tooth enamel. It's best to either avoid its use or brush your teeth shortly after chewing the tablet.

PARTNER NUTRIENTS: Used in conjunction with zinc, vitamin E, and beta-carotene, vitamin C has been shown to reduce vision loss from age-related macular degeneration. Vitamin C enhances the absorption of non-heme (plant-based) iron and chromium, and plays a role in activating folate.

SPECIAL POPULATIONS: We experience more oxidative stress as we age and since there is no harm with this dose of vitamin C and a big potential upside, I recommend people over the age of 50 take 200 mg of vitamin C two times daily, in addition to what is your multivitamin and diet. The most common inherited disease in the United States is hemochromatosis, a condition where the body has a strong genetic propensity to store iron. If your health-care provider has told you have this condition, not only do you need to avoid iron supplements but also should also limit the vitamin C in your supplements. (Read more about hemochromatosis under "Iron," page XX).

WARNING!
Don't Take Vitamin C When You're Going to Have Lab Tests

Vitamin C supplements of 1,000 mg or higher can interfere with numerous laboratory tests. Do not take more than 300 mg of supplemental vitamin C within 24 hours of testing.

VITAMIN D

Sir Edward Mellanby was a physician at King's College in London when he set upon the task of trying to find the cause of rickets, a disease that causes the softening and deformity of the bones, which was an all-too-common condition in the United Kingdom, particularly in Scotland. Thinking something in the diet must be responsible for the disease, he fed a group of dogs nothing but oatmeal, the main dietary staple among the Scots. Sure enough, the dogs all developed rickets. In 1919, Dr. Mellanby showed that he could cure the dogs by giving them cod liver oil, leading him to believe that rickets was due to a lack of vitamin A, a key component of cod liver oil. Cod liver oil was a highly effective treatment for rickets not because of its vitamin A, but because it is an excellent source of vitamin D, a fat-soluble vitamin that had yet to be discovered.

Although we call it a vitamin, vitamin D isn't really a vitamin at all. Vitamins are substances the body requires in small amounts that it cannot make and must be supplied in the daily diet. However, humans can make vitamin D following exposure to sunlight. Energy from the sun turns a chemical in our skin into previtamin D3, which is rapidly converted to vitamin D3 and either stored in fat cells or transported through our bloodstream to the liver, where it is converted to calcidiol, or 25(OH)D, the form we measure when we order a vitamin D test. Calcidiol must then travel to the kidneys, where it is converted to the biologically active calcitriol.

There are two primary forms of vitamin D: ergocalciferol (vitamin D2), which comes from yeast and is present in mushrooms, and cholecalciferol (vitamin D3), which is synthesized in the skin.

WHAT IT DOES: Vitamin D is critical for many functions in the body. From the story of rickets, we know that having adequate amounts is crucial for healthy bones. Working closely with parathyroid hormone (PTH), vitamin D controls calcium and phosphorous levels, which are necessary for strong bones, muscle contraction, nerve conduction, and the general function of all our cells. When calcium levels fall, the parathyroid gland secretes PTH, activating vitamin D, which increases intestinal absorption of calcium, and decreases excretion of calcium by the kidneys. However, if dietary calcium remains low, calcium is removed from the bone to maintain a constant supply in the bloodstream, which will eventually weaken them. You need calcium and vitamin D, and as I will explain later, vitamin K as well.

It might surprise you to know that the active form of vitamin D interacts with more than 30 different tissues in the body and affects more than 1,000 genes! In other words, it's important for a whole lot of things other than your bones! Vitamin D is necessary for maintaining muscle strength, which can help reduce the risk of falls and fractures. A meta-analysis of clinical trials published in the *British Medical Journal* in 2009 found that taking 700 to 1,000 IU per day of vitamin D3 lowered the risk of falls by 19 percent, while taking 200 to 600 IU per day offered no protection.

Vitamin D has a significant impact on the immune system. When it comes to autoimmune diseases, such as rheumatoid arthritis, multiple sclerosis, or lupus, vitamin D seems to act as an immunosuppressant, reducing flare-ups. Some evidence even suggests that vitamin D supplementation early in life may protect against diabetes. Research in Finland, following 10,000 children for over 30 years, showed that children who took vitamin D supplements in babyhood had a 90 percent lower risk of developing type 1 (insulin-dependent) diabetes, an autoimmune disorder that usually strikes before age 30.

Vitamin D increases our resistance to infections, particularly bacterial and viral infections that impact our respiratory tract. Studies suggest that people with low levels of vitamin D may be more likely to have more upper respiratory tract infections than those with normal levels. Interestingly, a 2015 study published in *Acta Pediatrica* found that getting enough vitamin D during pregnancy and early infancy reduced the number of primary care visits for the baby. A double-blinded study of 260 healthy pregnant women in New Zealand found that the babies of women who took 2,000 IU of vitamin D3 from 27 weeks' gestation to birth and then were given 800 IU per day of vitamin D3 for six months had a significantly lower incidence of acute respiratory infection compared to those who received a placebo.

This protective effect may be particularly important for people with asthma. While the findings are still somewhat preliminary, researchers are finding that vitamin D deficiency may be associated with increased airway hyperreactivity, worse asthma control, and possibly decreased response to standard asthma treatments. A study by researchers at Children's National Medical Center in Washington, D.C., found that African American youth (ages 6–20) with persistent asthma were significantly more likely to have low vitamin D when compared to controls. As the authors concluded, "Given the emerging associations between low vitamin D levels and asthma, strong consideration should be given to routine vitamin D testing in urban African American youth, particularly those with asthma." Further complicating the issue are the rates of obesity in this community: Obesity is also strongly associated with low vitamin D, worse asthma symptoms, and poor response to treatment. *Bottom line: If you have asthma, I strongly encourage you to have your vitamin D level checked and until then, to consider taking 1,000 to 2,000 IU per day of vitamin D3.*

There is some evidence that vitamin D may help protect us against colorectal cancer. Researchers from the National Cancer Institute evaluated vitamin D levels and colorectal cancer risk in the Prostate, Lung, Colorectal and Ovarian Cancer Screening Trial and found that higher levels of vitamin D were associated with a substantially lower risk for colorectal cancer. A 2014 meta-analysis published in the *European Journal of Cancer* found that higher 25(OH)D levels (>30 ng/mL) were associated with significantly reduced mortality in people with colorectal and breast cancer. The evidence for vitamin D and other cancers is inconsistent. *Bottom line: I recommend all cancer patients keep their vitamin D levels above 30 ng/mL. Talk to your oncologist about what your optimal range should be.*

Your heart contains vitamin D receptors as well, and vitamin D is important for maintaining healthy heart function and blood pressure. In the Health Professional Follow-Up Study, men with vitamin D deficiency were twice as likely to have a heart attack as men with adequate levels. A 2013 review of 21 studies in the *American Journal of Clinical Nutrition* found that vitamin D supplementation is protective against heart failure. While more research is needed, given that heart disease is the number one cause of death in the United States, making sure your vitamin D levels are normal is a smart idea.

FOOD SOURCES: The majority of dietary vitamin D in United States comes from the artificial fortification of milk or nondairy milk products, breakfast cereals, and orange juice. Herring, salmon (wild), sardines, and fish liver oils are good natural sources of vitamin D3. You can also get small amounts in eggs, beef, and butter.

SIGNS OF DEFICIENCY: Severe vitamin D deficiency during infancy or childhood leads to rickets, characterized by weak malformed bones, such as bowed legs and rib cage deformities, and seizures caused by very low levels of blood calcium. In adults, vitamin D deficiency causes osteomalacia, characterized by weak and painful muscles and bones, and increases the risk for osteoporosis. For the vast majority of people, mild deficiencies do not produce any overt signs but may increase our risk for heart disease, infections, and certain cancers.

RISK FOR DEFICIENCY: According to the CDC Second National Report on Biochemical Indicators of Diet and Nutrition in the U.S. Population, more than 66 million Americans have vitamin D insufficiency with 25(OH)D levels in the 12 to 20 ng/mL range, while 23 million are deficient with levels less than 12 ng/mL. A vitamin D level less than 12 ng/mL can lead to rickets in children and osteomalacia in adults. These are absolutely shocking numbers! And the number of people with insufficient levels is even higher if we use 30 ng/mL as the threshold for adequate levels as set by the Endocrine Society. Non-Hispanic blacks had the highest prevalence of low vitamin D levels (40 percent), followed by Mexican Americans (35 percent) and non-Hispanic whites (17 percent). Women were at greater risk than men for deficiency.

Why are we seeing such low levels of vitamin D? Compared to our ancestors, we spend more time indoors, wear more clothes, use sunscreen, live farther from the equator (at least, many of us do)—and the population is aging. Getting adequate sun exposure is the optimal way to maintain our vitamin D levels. People with very light skin may need only ten minutes three or four times per week, while those with very dark skin might need one to two hours to make the vitamin D they need. Darker pigments in the skin interfere with the ability of UV light to reach the layer of skin where vitamin D is produced. While sunscreen protects us against the damaging effects of UV radiation, an SPF of 8 blocks the production of vitamin D by a whopping 95 percent. The farther you live from the equator, the less UV light will be available for you to make vitamin D, particularly in the winter. As we age, our skin becomes thinner, making it more difficult for our skin cells to produce vitamin D. For all these reasons, taking a vitamin D supplement makes sense for all of us.

RDA/AI: Men under 70: 600 IU   Women under 70: 600 IU
After 70: 800 IU   After 70: 800 IU
Pregnancy: 600 IU
Breastfeeding: 600 IU

DV: 400 IU

UL: 4,000 IU (for ages 9 years and up)

SUPPLEMENT CONSIDERATIONS: It is hard to know how much vitamin D someone should take. It depends upon where you live, the color of your skin, how much time you spend outdoors, and your weight and diet, to name just a few variables. This is why I strongly encourage you to get your vitamin D level checked so you know exactly how much you need.

Our body uses cholecalciferol, or vitamin D3, which makes it the optimal form for supplementation. The vast majority of vitamin D3 in supplements is produced from either lanolin or fish liver oil. Ergocalciferol, or vitamin D2, is commercially prepared from ergosterol (present in yeast) and is generally preferred by vegans.

I recommend 2,000 IU per day of vitamin D3 for adults and 1,000 IU per day for kids and teens. The upper limit is 4,000 IU per day, so these recommendations are well within the "safe" range. Vitamin D is a fat-soluble vitamin that needs to be taken with some fat. Dinner tends to be richer in fat than other meals. One study found that taking vitamin D increased blood levels of vitamin D by 50 percent more than when it was taken with breakfast. *Bottom line: The optimal amount of vitamin D is the amount that gets your level at or above 30 ng/mL, which is why you should ask your health-care provider to order a vitamin D test or order it yourself! I generally try to keep my patient's levels around 35 ng/mL, or within the range of 30-50 ng/mL.*

PARTNER NUTRIENTS: Vitamin D works closely with calcium, magnesium, zinc and vitamin K to maintain bone health.

SPECIAL POPULATIONS: There is evidence that vitamin D can help prevent disease flare-ups in people with inflammatory bowel disease. Studies also suggest it can improve the symptoms of atopic dermatitis (eczema). I encourage anyone with either of these conditions to supplement with the doses I've recommended above. If you plan on becoming pregnant, have your vitamin D level checked and corrected first if possible. Studies show that having adequate vitamin D during pregnancy can be protective for both mom and baby. Newborn babies who are exclusively breastfed should be given 400 IU per day of vitamin D. To make sure the baby gets what she needs, just put one drop of vitamin D oil (400 IU) on your nipple and let the baby nurse. Alternate breasts each day. The vitamin D can also help prevent cracking and chafing of the nipple. Vegetarians and vegans need to take extra D2, which is less bioavailable than D3.

Warning:
Don't Exceed the RDA of Vitamin D
If You Have These Conditions

If you have hyperparathyroidism, Hodgkin's or non-Hodgkin's lymphoma, granulomatous disease (sarcoidosis, tuberculosis), kidney stones, kidney disease, or liver disease, make sure you talk to your health-care provider *before taking* more than the RDA of vitamin D.

VITAMIN E

In 1922, two physicians at the University of California, Berkeley, Herbert M. Evans and Katharine Scott Bishop, found that rats became sterile when fed a diet of butterfat, lard, cornstarch, casein, yeast, and salt. Feeding them wheat germ oil or lettuce resulted in the restoration of the rats' fertility. Evans and Bishop didn't know what compound in these foods was responsible for this effect, so they called it the "anti-sterility factor." In 1925, Evans decided to name this fifth vitamin "E," since the first four vitamins had been named A, B, C, and D. A colleague and professor of Greek literature proposed that he name it tocopherol, from the Greek *tokos,* meaning "offspring" and *phero,* meaning "to bear" for its critical role in reproduction. In 1969, the FDA recognized vitamin E as an essential nutrient for humans.

Naturally occurring vitamin E is actually a collection of eight fat-soluble antioxidants that include four tocopherols (alpha-, beta-, gamma-, delta-), and four tocotrienols (alpha-, beta-, gama-, delta-). Alpha-tocopherol is considered to be the most bioavailable form in the human body and it is the form that has been most widely studied.

WHAT IT DOES: Vitamin E is a powerhouse nutrient that helps maintain the health and function of the reproductive, vascular, and nervous systems, as well as our muscles. Because of its antioxidant activity, it was long thought that giving vitamin E supplements would reduce the risk of heart disease, but the data has generally shown negative results overall. There are some notable exceptions. In the large Women's Health Study, women aged 65 and older who took 600 IU of natural vitamin E every other day were found to have a significant reduction (26 percent) in heart attacks and dying from heart disease (49 percent), but there was no benefit to younger women. We know today that inflammation, more than even cholesterol, drives heart disease. A 2015 meta-analysis of clinical trials published in the *European Journal of Clinical Nutrition* found that natural vitamin E supplements in the form of alpha-tocopherol or gamma-tocopherol significantly reduced inflammation. This has important implications for the potential role for vitamin E in conditions other than heart disease: diabetes, arthritis, possibly even cancer.

We know that oxidative stress can lead to DNA damage, impairing cellular division and growth. This can be dangerous because DNA is the architect for cellular division; if the DNA is damaged, the abnormal cells can leave us vulnerable to cancer. Because of vitamin E's antioxidant activity, it was hoped that vitamin E might play a major role in preventing cancer. The American Cancer Society released the results of a long-term study of almost one million U.S. adults that found that those who regularly took 200 IU per day of vitamin E for more than 10 years had a lower risk of dying from bladder cancer. But another study, the SELECT trial, which was designed to determine if vitamin E, selenium, or the combination of the two could reduce the risk of prostate cancer in 35,000 men, found that there was statistically significant *increase* (17 percent) in prostate cancer in men taking 400 IU per day of vitamin E (d-alpha-tocopheryl acetate). Clearly, there is more work to be done to know the optimal form and dose, who might benefit and who may be at risk from taking supplemental vitamin E. *Bottom line: I wouldn't rely on vitamin E for general cancer prevention. However, if you've had bladder cancer, I would strongly encourage you to consider taking 200 IU per day of natural vitamin E.*

As we age, the brain becomes increasingly vulnerable to oxidative stress, which contributes to the development of dementia. With roughly 4.6 million new cases of dementia being diagnosed every year, the search is on for interventions that can slow the process. Studies suggest vitamin E may delay cognitive decline in people with mild forms of Alzheimer's disease. The Trial of Vitamin E and Memantine in Alzheimer's Disease: Veterans Affairs [VA] Cooperative Randomized Trial was a large double-blinded, placebo-controlled study of 613 veterans with mild-to-moderate Alzheimer's dementia (AD) being treated at numerous VA medical centers. Participants were given either

1,000 IU of dl-alpha tocopheryl acetate (synthetic vitamin E) twice daily, 10 mg of memantine (an FDA approved drug for dementia) twice daily, the combination of both, or placebo. The duration of treatment ranged from six months to four years. The results were published in the *Journal of the American Medical Association* in 2014. Taking vitamin E resulted in slower functional decline (19 percent) compared to placebo, while neither memantine alone or with vitamin E showed any meaningful clinical benefit. This high dose of vitamin E was well tolerated and there were no safety issues. The results of this study confirmed an earlier trial in people with moderate to severe AD that showed similar findings. *Bottom line: If you have a loved one dealing with early cognitive decline or Alzheimer's, talk to that person's health-care provider about this study and see if this treatment would be appropriate.*

Some women report that higher doses of vitamin E (600–800 IU per day) improve their hot flashes and fibrocystic breast disease. While I believe individual women might experience benefit, clinical trials don't show any significant benefit in taking vitamin E for either condition. I do, however, often recommend vitamin E suppositories for vaginal dryness in women who can't take estrogen. Vitamin E is also important for the reproductive health of men, supporting the proper structure and functioning of sperm. Several studies have found that vitamin E supplementation helps improve male fertility.

A growing number of adults and children in the US have non-alcoholic steatohepatitis (NASH), a condition where fats build up in the liver, causing inflammation and damage. It is similar to the liver disease caused by long-term, heavy drinking, but NASH occurs in people who don't abuse alcohol. Risk factors include obesity, diabetes, insulin resistance, and metabolic syndrome. (I think you can understand why we're seeing more of it these days!)

In 2015, the *Journal of Gastroenterology* concluded that vitamin E is an evidence-based treatment option for this condition. Studies have shown that taking 800 IU per day of vitamin E for 24 months significantly improved liver enzymes, fatty infiltration of the liver, and liver inflammation. The big question is not so much is it effective, but is vitamin E safe at this dose over an extended period of time?

And last, but not least, vitamin E is important for healthy skin, hair, and nails, explaining why it is found in numerous skin creams and lotions. Vitamin E is often used to help promote wound healing and prevent scarring, but there really isn't any evidence to support this practice. A couple of small postsurgical studies failed to show any significant beneficial effect.

FOOD SOURCES: Vitamin E is abundant in sunflower seeds. One tablespoon contains roughly 10 IU, so make sure to add some to your diet—they taste great in salad! Almonds, spinach, avocados, green leafy vegetables, vegetable oils, wheat germ, fatty fish, and eggs are also good sources. Alpha-tocopherol is abundant in olive oil, which is why it is the predominant form in the European diet. On the other hand, gamma-tocopherol is abundant in soybean and corn oil, making it the most common form in the American diet.

SIGNS OF DEFICIENCY: There are no obvious signs or symptoms that accompany mild vitamin E deficiency. With prolonged deficiency, there is an increased risk for peripheral neuropathy, infection, anemia, and poor pregnancy outcomes for both the mother and the baby.

RISK FOR DEFICIENCY: According to the Office of Dietary Supplements at the National Institutes of Health, "The diets of most Americans provide less than the recommended amounts of vitamin E." Very low fat diets can put you at risk for deficiency, as can any disease or disorder that causes a problem with fat absorption such as cystic fibrosis or Crohn's disease.

RDA/AI: Men: 15 mg (22.4 IU)   Women: 15 mg (22.4 IU)
Pregnancy: 15 mg (22.4 IU)
Breastfeeding: 19 mg
(28.4 IU)

DV: 30 IU

UL: 1,500 IU of natural vitamin E and 1,100 IU of synthetic vitamin E

SUPPLEMENT CONSIDERATIONS: A multivitamin that provides 30 IU of vitamin E is probably adequate for most of us. I generally discourage people from taking more than 100 IU per day of natural vitamin E long-term, unless it is for a specific condition, as there have not been *any* adverse events associated with this level of intake. Make sure you look to see what kind of vitamin E it is, because this is one instance where synthetic is not as good as natural. Vitamin E listed, as dl-alpha-tocopherol or dl-alpha-tocopheryl acetate is synthetic and only one-half as bioavailable as the natural d-alpha-tocopherol. Some experts recommend supplements that provide the full complement of all eight antioxidant forms of vitamin E. Vitamin E supplements should be taken with a meal that contains some fat, for best absorption.

PARTNER NUTRIENTS: Optimal use of vitamin E is dependent on selenium, copper, zinc, and manganese. Vitamin E is needed to protect vitamin A from oxidation in the body.

SPECIAL POPULATIONS: People with Crohn's disease, cystic fibrosis, and a rare genetic disorder called abetalipoproteinemia are at substantially increased risk for vitamin E deficiency, making supplementation a necessity.

VITAMIN K

Henrik Dam, a Danish researcher, found that when he fed chickens a cholesterol-free diet, they had a tendency to bleed. He then discovered that he could reverse this condition if he fed them alfalfa, spinach, cabbage, or liver. Dam deduced that the disease was caused by a deficiency of a substance that helped thicken the blood. He named it vitamin K for the German word *Koagulation* (coagulation). In 1939, he and the American researcher Edward Doisy, working independently, isolated vitamin K from alfalfa. They shared the 1943 Nobel Prize for Medicine. Today, we know that vitamin K is essential for far more than blood clotting.

Vitamin K is actually three fat-soluble vitamins: vitamin K1 (phylloquinone or phytonadione), vitamin K2 (menaquinone), and vitamin K3 (menadione). K1 is highest in leafy green vegetables, with very small amounts present in dairy, while K2 is found in fermented foods, such as natto, sauerkraut, and cheese, as well as egg yolks, butter from grass-fed cows, chicken liver and breast, and ground beef. K3 (menadione) is a synthetic form of vitamin K. The body is capable of converting K1 to K2.

WHAT IT DOES: It's well known that vitamin K is critically important for ensuring that our blood clots when needed, so I want to spend a little time talking about its potential role in cardiovascular and bone health, and possibly in cancer—beneficial effects that fewer people are aware of. The story begins with the so-called calcium paradox, a term originally coined when researchers observed that some postmenopausal women taking calcium supplements had increasing arterial calcification with a simultaneous *loss* of bone mineral density. In other words, in some women, it appeared as if the supplemental calcium was failing to get into the bones where it was needed most and was instead accumulating in the walls of blood vessels. The missing link might be vitamin K, or vitamin K2 specifically, which acts like a traffic cop for calcium, directing it towards the bones and teeth and away from tissues where it doesn't belong, such as the blood vessels. Vitamin K2 activates matrix Gla-protein (MGP), a potent inhibitor of arterial and soft tissue calcification.

The Rotterdam study, a 10-year prospective study that gathered dietary and other data on 7,983 men and women over 55 years of age in the Netherlands, added key information. Stunningly, results published in the *Journal of Nutrition* showed high dietary intake of K2, but not K1, had a strong protective effect on cardiovascular health. Eating foods rich in natural vitamin K2 (at least 32 mcg per day) resulted in a 50 percent reduction in arterial calcification and death due to cardiovascular disease. Wow! This study was fascinating in no small part because the foods providing K2 were meat, eggs, and cheese—not often considered part of a heart healthy diet! The intake of phylloquinone (K1) in this study was 250 mcg/day, higher than in the U.S. population aged 55 and over, where intakes are 80 to 210 mcg/d—but it seemed to have very little effect on heart disease. The Rotterdam trial is consistent with other studies that have shown a consistent reduction in coronary artery calcification with vitamin K2.

Let's look at the role of vitamin K in bone health. The Nurses' Health Study and the Framingham Heart Study, two famous longitudinal studies, have shown that people with low dietary intake of vitamin K have a greater risk of fractures, including hip fractures. In part, this is because vitamin K is required for the carboxylation, or activation, of an important bone-building protein called osteocalcin. Studies show that when osteocalcin is undercarboxylated, it more than doubles the risk of hip fracture in women. Studies have shown that both K1 and K2 increase the carboxylation of osteocalcin. A study of 100 healthy adults showed that those who took vitamin K1 supplements for two weeks had better activation of osteocalcin, meaning their bones were taking in more calcium than the bones of those receiving placebo or lower doses. The research shows that vitamins D and K, along with calcium and a host of other minerals, are all important when it comes to maintaining strong bones.

If this isn't enough to get you excited about vitamin K, the findings from the *European Prospective Investigation into Cancer and Nutrition (EPIC-Heidelberg cohort)* might: They show that men with the highest dietary intakes of K2 had a 35 percent lower risk of prostate cancer! The study enrolled and followed 25,540 men (40–64 years old) and women (35–64 years old) who were initially free of cancer, for more than 10 years. The findings, published in the *American Journal of Clinical Nutrition*, also reported that the highest intake of K2 reduced the risk of lung cancer by 62 percent. More research is needed before we fully understand the relationship between vitamin K and cancer, however this preliminary research is very intriguing.

FOOD SOURCES: Dark green leafy vegetables are the main food source of vitamin K1. One cup of kale provides 1,000 mcg of K1, the level needed to lower undercarboxylated osteocalcin levels and strengthen bones! Other vegetables, such as spinach, mustard greens, turnip greens, Swiss chard, lettuce, and broccoli, as well as avocado and kiwi fruits, can also help keep your vitamin K levels where they need to be. Including some soft and hard cheese and eggs (with the yolks, please) can ramp up your vitamin K2 levels. Fermented foods are also a good source of K2. Natto is a Japanese dish made from fermented soybeans and while some might find it an "acquired taste," it is a very good vegetarian source of K2.

SIGNS OF DEFICIENCY: Vitamin K deficiency causes symptoms such as bleeding gums, frequent nose bleeds, easy bruising, and, if you're female, heavy menstrual periods.

RISK FOR DEFICIENCY: More people may have marginal vitamin K levels due to the lack of regular vegetable consumption. Alcoholics are at higher risk for vitamin K deficiency, as is anyone with a digestive disorder that impairs the absorption of fats (Crohn's disease, cystic fibrosis, etc.).

RDA/AI: Men: 120 mcg/day   Women: 90 mcg/day

DV: 80 mcg

UL: None set. There has not been any reported toxicity associated with high intakes of vitamin K. Taking high doses of vitamin K will *not* increase your risk for blood clots.

SUPPLEMENT CONSIDERATIONS: If you are eating a healthy diet rich in vitamin K foods, then taking a multivitamin with 150 to 300 mcg per day of K1 is a good target. Given the potential benefit and very low risk, supplementing with 500 mcg of vitamin K2, preferably as MK-4, seems reasonable if you have cardiovascular disease, diabetes, are at risk for osteoporosis, or are concerned about prostate cancer. (Note about vitamin K2: It has a number of subtypes and the two that are of the most interest in human health are MK-4 and MK-7.)

> # *WARNING!*
> ## Don't Mix Vitamin K Supplements
> ## with Warfarin
> If you are taking warfarin (Coumadin) to prevent blood clots,
> do not exceed the RDA for vitamin K.

PARTNER NUTRIENTS: As mentioned earlier, vitamin K partners with vitamin D and calcium, as well as magnesium and zinc. Large doses of vitamin A can interfere with the absorption of vitamin K.

SPECIAL POPULATIONS: Vitamin K deficiency in a newborn can lead to a serious bleeding disorder, called hemorrhagic disease of the newborn (HDN). Babies can be at increased risk for HDN if they are born prematurely, are low birth weight, were delivered by C-section or with the use of forceps—or if the labor was extremely fast or prolonged. An intramuscular vitamin K1 injection is typically given after birth to protect against both early and late vitamin K deficiency bleeding. Some parents prefer to use an oral solution, but if you choose to do so, and are breastfeeding, it's absolutely critical to give it as directed by your pediatrician for the full three months.

So now you know the vital facts about vitamins, and how to be sure you are getting enough but not too much given your unique health profile. A high-quality multivitamin is your best supplement seatbelt, but now you know which other vitamins you might need to look for in the supplement aisle. Next, we'll look at minerals, in which you might also be deficient.

Chapter 4

Minerals

Like vitamins, minerals are absolutely essential for your health. Your body is unable to manufacture any of these minerals, so they must be obtained in your diet. Some minerals, such as calcium and magnesium, are needed in large quantities, whereas others, such as selenium or chromium, require only trace amounts. Minerals are critically important for a wide variety of functions in the body: helping muscles to contract and relax, producing stomach acid, maintaining healthy bones and teeth, regulating blood pressure and heart rhythm, transporting oxygen to cells, making thyroid hormones, and so much more.

In this chapter I would like to focus on the minerals that I believe are critically important for your health, those that are at commonly deficient in the American diet and those that are often found in dietary supplements. It doesn't mean that molybdenum, sulfur, sodium, chloride, manganese, and phosphorous aren't important—they are! Let's look at those minerals more closely. Sodium chloride is salt, and we get plenty of that in our diet. There is no evidence of molybdenum deficiency in the

U.S. The concern with manganese is not generally deficiency but the risk of toxicity from excess. Phosphorous is very common in the American diet. It is plentiful in protein-rich foods (meat, fish, poultry, eggs, dairy, nuts, beans), whole grains, and carbonated beverages. When calcium levels are low, your body excretes phosphorous in the urine, which plays a critical role in bone health. So, while it is possible to have low phosphorous levels, getting too much in our diet is far more common than having too little.

The only one of these minerals that might be of concern is sulfur, as it is vitally important for the liver to undertake its detoxification processes. Proteins are the best sources of sulfur and studies show that Americans are getting plenty: 70 grams per day for adult women and over 100 grams per day for adult men. However, elders and vegans may have marginal protein intake, so taking a dietary supplement containing organic sulfur might be reasonable.

The minerals that are critically important for our well-being *and* in which we are likely to be deficient are calcium, chromium, iodine, iron, magnesium, potassium, selenium, and zinc. As in the chapter about vitamins, I'll go through each one and share with you what science shows and what I know from personal and professional experience.

CALCIUM

Calcium is a soft, gray metal found in the bones and teeth of humans and animals in the form of calcium salts. It's also found in seashells and limestone—in fact, the word *calcium* comes from a Latin root meaning "lime." *Most of us know that calcium is fundamental for having healthy bones and teeth, but calcium is actually used by almost every cell in our body.* Calcium helps muscles contract, blood clot, cells communicate with each other, the heart maintain a regular beat, blood pressure stay within a normal range, secretion of insulin and other hormones, and much more.

Unquestionably, this mineral is incredibly vital to our overall health. It is especially important for adolescents who are growing rapidly and building strong bones. Teens are the ones who need calcium the most and are often the ones who don't get it; however, in my experience it's mostly older women who are loading up on calcium. I routinely see 55-year-old women taking 600 mg of calcium supplements twice a day, with another 200 mg in their multivitamin, on top of getting 1,000 mg per day in their diet. That's 2,400 mg per day! The upper tolerable limit for *all* sources of calcium for someone over the age of 50 is 2,000 mg! This high intake of calcium is not necessary and may actually be harmful.

WHAT IT DOES: Calcium is the most abundant mineral in our body, with roughly 99 percent of it stored in our teeth and bones. Bones act as a storage reservoir for calcium, where it helps maintain the integrity of our skeleton. If calcium is needed elsewhere, it is taken from the bones. This is why you want to make sure you're getting adequate amounts in your diet. The more you have to remove the calcium you've stored in your bones, the weaker your bones will become over time. From childhood through elder years, both men and women need to ensure they are getting enough calcium, along with vitamins D and K, magnesium, trace minerals, regular exercise, and protein to build and then maintain healthy bones and teeth. The other one percent of the body's calcium is found in our bloodstream and soft tissues where it plays an important role in many biological processes:

A dysregulation of calcium may contribute to premenstrual symptoms. Studies have shown women with higher dietary intake of calcium have fewer PMS symptoms, and several studies have shown that calcium supplementation (500–600 mg two times per day) reduces mood swings, irritability, breast tenderness, and sugar cravings. A 2009 review in the *Canadian Journal of Clinical Pharmacology* concluded that calcium has good-quality evidence to support its use in PMS.

Calcium helps regulate the constriction and relaxation of blood vessels, which is why it may help prevent high blood pressure, particularly in those who are sensitive to salt or have low dietary calcium. A 2006 review of thirteen studies by the international Cochrane Group found that calcium has a modest effect on systolic blood pressure (the top number) but no effect on diastolic blood pressure. The beneficial effect of calcium on blood pressure, however, may be particularly important during pregnancy. A review by the Cochrane Group that included 15,730 pregnant women found that supplementing with at least 1,000 mg per day of calcium starting at approximately 20 weeks of pregnancy (34 weeks at the latest) significantly reduced the risk of high blood pressure and preeclampsia—a condition that involves a rapid spike in blood pressure during the last trimester accompanied by swelling and protein in the urine, which can be life-threatening to mother and baby if left untreated.

While public health initiatives have greatly reduced our exposure to lead, even low levels can increase the risk of premature birth and are dangerous to the brain and nervous system of babies in the womb and during early childhood. A study of the drinking water from 63 elementary schools in Seattle, Washington, and 601 elementary schools in Los Angeles, California, found that even after corrective measures (installing water filters and removing lead pipes), around 5 percent of these schoolchildren in Seattle and 6 percent in Los Angeles still exceeded the safe blood levels of lead. Calcium protects against lead toxicity by reducing the amount of lead absorbed in the GI tract and preventing it from being released from the skeleton, where it is stored. A study by Harvard researchers found that when pregnant women received either 1,200 mg per day of calcium or placebo beginning in their first trimester, the women who took calcium had 11 percent lower levels of lead in their blood compared to the women who took the placebo. Similar reductions in lead levels in breast milk were noted in women taking supplemental calcium. And after menopause, as women lose bone mineral density, the lead that was long stored in the skeleton begins to move into the bloodstream.

There are studies that suggest that calcium may help protect us against colorectal cancer and may help us maintain a healthy body weight. And if all these benefits of calcium weren't enough, calcium carbonate is FDA approved for the occasional treatment of heartburn because it acts as a buffering agent, reducing acidity in the stomach that can cause heartburn. Calcium is also necessary for the absorption of vitamin B12. Preliminary research shows that calcium may help prevent the B12 depletion that occurs secondary to taking the diabetes drug metformin (Glucophage).

WHAT TO EAT: Dairy foods, such as cheese, yogurt, and milk, provide most of the calcium in the American diet. Ample supplies are also found in firm tofu as well as fortified soy milk and orange juice. And for those of you who don't like milk or soy, the calcium found in vegetables that belong to the kale family (broccoli, cabbage, bok choy, mustard, and turnip greens) is every bit as bioavailable as the calcium in dairy. Dried apricots and almonds are also good sources of absorbable calcium. Spinach is loaded in calcium but it is also high in oxalate, which interferes with calcium absorption, making only about 10 percent of its calcium available to the body for use.

SIGNS OF DEFICIENCY: One of the first signs of calcium deficiency is often muscle cramping. Muscle aches of the thighs and arms with minimal exertion could indicate a deficiency of calcium, vitamin D, and/or magnesium. Many of the signs—such as numbness or tingling of the fingers, poor appetite, and fatigue—are fairly nonspecific and could indicate a host of things. Extreme calcium deficiency in childhood, just like vitamin D deficiency, can cause rickets, a condition where the bones are soft and bow outward, causing bowleggedness.

RISK FOR DEFICIENCY: Those with low dietary calcium intake are at greatest risk for deficiency, as are those with specific medical conditions, such as epilepsy, autoimmune disease, and heart failure; primarily because many of the medications used to treat these disorders deplete the body of calcium.

Pregnant women should be vigilant about getting enough calcium to reduce their risk of preeclampsia and make certain that their baby's bones develop properly. Children and teens are building bone rapidly and experiencing growth spurts, so their calcium needs are high. Remember, we only build bone until our mid-20s, so we have a limited window of time during which to build the strong bones and teeth needed to carry us through the rest of our lives.

Teenagers, who need calcium the most, generally have the least in their diet compared to children and adults. As many kids have swapped their glass of milk for a can of soda, I suggest parents be very diligent about ensuring their children and teens are getting plenty of calcium!

Consuming more than 300 mg per day of caffeine (3–4 cups of coffee, or six 12-ounce sodas) can increase the urinary excretion of calcium. While this sounds bad, the overall effect is relatively small. For every cup of coffee, there is about a 2 to 3 mg loss of calcium. If you enjoy your coffee, just make sure you are including plenty of calcium rich foods.

Sodium is the other robber of calcium. It takes 1,000 mg of calcium per day to maintain calcium balance for every 2,000 mg per day of sodium. Folks, 1 teaspoon of salt contains 2,300 mg of sodium! A diet rich in potassium helps counter the ill effects of sodium but many Americans are also low in this important mineral. *Bottom line: Eat a potassium-rich diet, ensure you are getting adequate calcium in your diet, and keep your salt intake to roughly 1 teaspoon per day (iodized, please!).*

Finally, low calcium levels are often associated with low blood levels of magnesium and vitamin D. These partner nutrients are essential for maintaining normal calcium levels in the body.

RDA/AI: Men 19–70: 1,000 mg
After 70: 1,200 mg

Women 19–50: 1,000 mg
After 50: 1,200 mg
Pregnancy: 1,000 mg
Breastfeeding: 1,000 mg

DV: 1,000 mg/day

UL: 2,500 mg/day is the upper limit for adults aged 19 to 50, and 2,000 mg per day for those over 50 years of age. Excessive intake of calcium is not good for you: It may increase the risk of fractures, prostate cancer, kidney stones, and heart disease. All that extra calcium has to go somewhere and you don't need it settling in where it doesn't belong. *Bottom line: Make sure you* *calculate how much calcium you are getting in your diet and supplement only the difference.*

FROM DR. LOW DOG

℞ Calcium Calculator: A Quick Estimate

Food	# Servings/ Day	Estimated Calcium per Serving, in mg	Calcium in mg
Milk (8 ounces)		× 300	=
Yogurt (6 ounces)		× 300	=
Hard cheese (1 ounce)		× 200	=
Soy milk, fortified (8 ounces)		× 300	=
Orange juice, fortified (8 ounces)		× 300	=
Tofu, firm, calcium set (4 ounces)		× 300	=
All calcium-rich foods not included above		× 250	=
		Total calcium	=
AI for your gender and age group		Subtract your total calcium from AI	= Supplement this amount

SUPPLEMENT CONSIDERATIONS: After you have calculated how much calcium you need to close the gap between what you are consuming in your diet and how much you require based upon your age and gender, you will need to find the right calcium supplement. There are several forms available. Keep in mind that elemental calcium comes attached to another compound, such as carbonate or citrate, and that compound can impact your ability to use the calcium.

The cheapest and most concentrated form of calcium (meaning you can take fewer pills) is calcium carbonate. You must take it with meals to ensure absorption—and it can be constipating. Now, if you are over the age of 50, taking acid-blocking medications, or have a history of kidney stones, calcium citrate is your best bet. It has less elemental calcium, meaning you have to take more pills than calcium carbonate to get the same dose, but it doesn't have to be taken with meals and is less likely to cause intestinal gas or constipation. Calcium citrate-malate is another combination that is widely available in dietary supplements and is well absorbed. Calcium gluconate, calcium lactate, and calcium phosphate have very low levels of calcium, and you'd have to take a handful of pills to get what you need. As for coral calcium—skip it. There are more environmentally friendly ways to get your calcium, so leave the coral alone!

Calcium can't be absorbed in large quantities. Don't supplement with more than 500 mg at a time. (*Note:* Most of you shouldn't be supplementing with more than 500 mg, anyway!) Some calcium pills can be hard to swallow because of their size, so you might want to try a chewable supplement. When my daughter was a young teenager, I kept a bowl of chocolate-, orange-, and caramel-flavored calcium supplements in a bowl so that she could pick one out to have after dinner. One 500 mg calcium chewable was enough to get her to the 1,300 milligrams she needed each day.

You need vitamins D and K, magnesium, zinc, and a whole host of other trace minerals to properly use your calcium. Remember, large doses of calcium can impair the absorption of trace minerals. The small amount of calcium in most multivitamin-mineral supplements won't interfere with absorption of other minerals, including iron and zinc. However, if you're taking 500 mg of calcium (the common amount in most calcium supplements), take your multivitamin, iron, or zinc at least two hours apart from your calcium.

PARTNER NUTRIENTS: Calcium in conjunction with vitamins D and K, magnesium, potassium, zinc and other trace minerals is vitally important for bone health. I want to stress that vitamin D, magnesium, and calcium are partners, working together to regulate parathyroid hormone and maintain stable levels of blood calcium. If you are deficient in vitamin D or magnesium, it can effect calcium regulation in the body. Focusing only on calcium without ensuring adequate intake of other nutrients is not a good idea.

SPECIAL POPULATIONS: When I was in medical school, one of my attending physicians told us, "Osteoporosis is a disease of childhood that manifests in old age." What he was trying to stress is that we only have a small window of time in which to fortify the skeleton for later years: You have to build the bone you need for the rest of your life by the time you are roughly 25 years old. While menopausal women, who are likely more health conscious than your average teen, may be going overboard with calcium supplements, their teenage children are skipping the multivitamin, drinking soda, and eating far too much salty food, and spending a lot of time indoors looking at screens instead of outdoors playing in the sun. All of this is a bad setup for future bone health, as well as bad for overall health now! Teens need roughly 1,300 mg of calcium every day!

Women with low BMIs (body mass index, the ratio of fat to weight), particularly female athletes, often have low levels of estrogen as estrogen levels are affected by body fat levels. With less estrogen, over time, they can lose bone mass. Female athletes who are of childbearing age and not having regular menstrual periods need to be especially diligent about getting enough calcium and vitamin D.

Some studies suggest that men who have the highest intakes of dairy and/or calcium in their diets are at greater risk for developing prostate cancer; other studies have found no link whatsoever. For instance, in a 10-year follow-up, researchers at Dartmouth Medical School found that when 672 men were given 1,200 mg per day of elemental calcium for four years, there was no increased risk of prostate cancer; indeed, there may have been a mild protective effect. Men should aim for getting a total of 1,000 mg per day of calcium (diet and supplements combined) until we know more about its possible relationship to prostate cancer.

CHROMIUM

Interest in chromium for the management of diabetes began more than 60 years ago when scientists found that feeding brewer's yeast to animals could prevent diabetes. Researchers postulated that the yeast contained a specific glucose tolerance factor (GTF). Even though the mineral chromium had been identified in the late 1700s, it wasn't until the 1970s that scientists discovered that this GTF factor in yeast was chromium and that it is essential for carbohydrate metabolism. With the increase of type 2 diabetes, more people are turning to chromium in the belief it will help keep their blood sugar levels stable.

Chromium is a common element in seawater and in the earth's crust. Our body requires only trace amounts. Chromium exists primarily in two forms: trivalent (chromium 3+), the biologically active form found in food, and hexavalent (chromium 6+), which is used and produced in industrial processes and can be highly toxic. We will be discussing only trivalent chromium.

Small amounts of chromium can be found in numerous foods, but processing lowers levels that might already be low from foods grown in chromium depleted soil. Vitamin C and certain

B-vitamins are needed to absorb chromium in the gut, nutrients that are often low in our diet.

WHAT IT DOES: Chromium is vital to the function of insulin, the pancreatic hormone that orchestrates the use of fuels from carbohydrates, fats, and protein. When blood sugar levels rise, the pancreas secretes insulin, which drives the sugar (glucose) out of the blood and into cells where it can be used for energy. Chromium enhances the action of insulin, increasing insulin sensitivity and the uptake of blood sugar by our cells. A deficiency of chromium in the diet may increase the risk of insulin resistance and predispose a person to obesity and type 2 diabetes.

RX FROM DR. LOW DOG
Two Primary Types of Diabetes

Because the research on chromium has been primarily on type 2 diabetes, it's important to understand the distinction between the two primary types of diabetes. In type 1, or "insulin-dependent," diabetes, which usually appears before age 30, immune cells destroy the cells in the pancreas that manufacture insulin, making insulin injections necessary. Type 2 diabetes can affect people of any age and is much more common in those who are overweight and sedentary. Initially, the problem is not with the pancreas but with the body's cells that are not able to efficiently take up the sugar (glucose) in our bloodstream. The pancreas responds by making more insulin in an attempt to force the sugar into the cells. This condition is called insulin resistance, or prediabetes. Over time, the pancreas is unable to make enough insulin to keep the blood sugar levels normal and the person often requires medication.

As mentioned earlier, the potential role of chromium in diabetes was first identified in the late 1950s, when researchers found that rats fed brewers' yeast were better able to maintain blood sugar stability. The key ingredient in brewer's yeast responsible for this effect was chromium. Since then, scientists have been looking at the potential role of chromium for preventing and treating diabetes. Unfortunately, the studies have yielded inconsistent results. Some studies show that it can lower blood sugar when taken at doses higher than 200 mcg per day, but others failed to show a lowering of hemoglobin A1C, the blood test that assesses someone's average blood sugar levels over the previous 90 days. The inconsistency in research results may be due to (1) the form of chromium was not optimal (yeast seems to best), (2) doses were often insufficient (200 mcg or less has not shown benefit), and/or (3) there is no readily available test to determine chromium levels. It's unclear if participants in the study were actually deficient in chromium and, if so, whether the deficiency was corrected with the dose and product used.

Some research has shown that chromium can lower triglycerides and raise HDL in people with high cholesterol, atherosclerosis (hardening of the arteries, caused by the buildup of plaque), or taking beta-blockers. Again, however, not all studies show benefit.

While chromium is often found in weight-loss products or those designed to increase muscle and decrease fat, if there is a benefit, it's small. However, some research suggests that supplemental chromium may reduce food cravings in overweight/obese women and in people with binge eating disorders when taken at a dose of 1,000 mcg per day.

WHAT TO EAT: The level of chromium in plant foods varies considerably based upon the soil they were grown in and how they were processed. Brewer's yeast (dried *Saccharomyces cerevisiae*) is one of the richest sources of biologically active chromium, GTF, containing around 60 mcg per tablespoon. Meat, whole grains, broccoli, green beans, tomatoes, nuts, and eggs are other good sources of chromium. Many people eat foods high in added sugars (sucrose and fructose), which are not only low in chromium but also increase its excretion from the body.

SIGNS OF DEFICIENCY: Even mild chromium deficiency can lead to problems in regulating our blood sugar, which over time may lead to the development of diabetes. Deficiency might also contribute to altered cholesterol metabolism, contributing to heart disease.

RISK FOR DEFICIENCY: Many of us may be at risk for mild deficiencies of chromium due to low soil levels of chromium and our overconsumption of highly refined and processed foods that enhance its excretion from the body.

Anyone with absorption problems due to medication use or such diseases as Crohn's disease may be low in chromium. While chromium can be stored—in the bone, liver, spleen, and soft tissues—our absorption of it is poor. Plus, we can lose chromium when we are under stress, eat lots of sugar, have an infection, or experience physical trauma.

Aerobic exercise causes the body to excrete chromium, whereas weight training increases absorption.

RDA/AI: Men 19–50: 35 mcg   Women 19–50: 25 mcg
After 50: 30 mcg   After 50: 20 mcg
Pregnancy: 30 mcg
Breastfeeding: 45 mcg

DV: 120 mcg

UL: Not determined. *Note:* Just because there isn't an upper limit doesn't mean that you should consider large doses of chromium safe. There simply isn't enough research to know where to set the upper limit. *I would caution against using more than 1,000 mcg per day.*

SUPPLEMENT CONSIDERATIONS: As you can see, the daily value of 120 mcg for chromium is higher than the RDA and is probably the right amount for most of us. While we await a large randomized trial to answer the question of whether supplemental chromium benefits people living with diabetes, a 90-day trial of 600 mcg per day of GTF chromium is reasonable and safe.

Chromium supplements come in several forms: chromium combined with picolinate, nicotinate, polynicotinate, or chloride. Chromium chloride is the least absorbed form, whereas picolinate or nicotinate enhance chromium absorption and retention in the body. Chromium picolinate is the most popular form and while considered safe, there are some suggestions that large doses (1,000 mcg per day or higher) might damage DNA. I prefer chromium derived from brewer's yeast, as it is the most bioavailable. Look on the label for chromium GTF.

PARTNER NUTRIENTS: One study that combined 600 mcg per day of chromium picolinate with 2 mg of biotin found that it improved blood glucose and cholesterol in type 2 diabetics. Chromium absorption is improved when it is paired with vitamin C.

SPECIAL POPULATIONS: Runners and other athletes, those with absorption problems, and anyone with insulin resistance or type 2 diabetes may want to consider chromium supplementation. In hereditary hemochromatosis, a genetic disorder that causes iron to build up in the body, chromium transport is impaired, which may explain why people with this condition often develop diabetes.

IODINE

Iodine is an essential nonmetallic trace element that exists in nature as elemental iodine or iodide. Iodide is simply iodine bound to another element, such as potassium or sodium. Iodine is absolutely critical for the production of thyroid hormones, and iodine deficiency is the leading cause of hypothyroidism in the world. It can be difficult to get iodine from our food. Seaweeds provide an excellent source, but they are not a typical staple in the American diet. When it comes to foods grown on land, iodine levels are dramatically impacted by soil quality and climate. As iodine levels are highest in the oceans, coastal soils tend to have higher levels than soils found farther inland.

You may not know this but iodine deficiency is the most preventable cause of brain damage in the world. In 1993, the World Health Organization (WHO) urged that salt iodization be adopted globally. Salt makes a great vehicle for delivering iodine as it is widely available and people tend to use it in similar amounts throughout the year. It's also very inexpensive, costing about a nickel per person per year. However, even with these enormous global health initiatives, according to the WHO, iodine deficiency remains one of the main causes of impaired cognitive development in children. The WHO estimates that over 30 percent of the world's population, or roughly 2.3 billion people, do not get sufficient iodine in their diets.

Earlier in the book I explained why we began adding iodine to salt in the U.S. It was to prevent goiter, a swelling of the thyroid that can occur due to iodine deficiency. For decades it was assumed that the U.S. was an iodine sufficient country, but new research shows that certain segments of our population may still be at risk for iodine deficiency, which should concern us all.

WHAT IT DOES: Iodine's most important role in the body is the production of thyroid hormones, which are crucial for maintaining body temperature, metabolism, and cellular growth. There are two primary thyroid hormones named for how many iodine molecules they contain: T4 has four iodine molecules and T3 (the most biologically active form of thyroid hormone) has three.

Thyroid hormones are manufactured in your thyroid gland located in the lower front of your neck. To produce them, you need to consume iodine, which is absorbed in the gastrointestinal tract and then transported to the thyroid gland as iodide. When the body is in need of thyroid hormone, the cells in the thyroid gland take up iodide via a pump called the sodium-iodide symporter.

Iodine concentrations are 20 to 40 times higher in the thyroid than in the bloodstream, but some of our body's iodine can be also be found in tissues, such as the breast, cervix, lungs, stomach, and salivary glands. Low levels of iodine in salivary glands may reduce the production of saliva, leaving you with a dry mouth. Two studies found that supplemental iodine is beneficial in treating fibrocystic breast disease. However, doses of 3,000-6,000 mcg per day were required to decrease breast pain, tenderness, and nodularity. That's a pretty hefty dose! There is some speculation that iodine may play a role in the prevention of breast cancer and stomach cancer. In the lungs, iodine improves our antiviral defenses.

Getting adequate iodine throughout our lives is important. During pregnancy, thyroid hormones are necessary for nerve and brain development in the baby. Myelin is the protective coating on our nerves that allows them to conduct signals effectively, and thyroid hormone is responsible for myelination of a baby's developing nervous system. Because we need iodine to produce thyroid hormone, iodine deficiency during pregnancy can be harmful, causing stillbirth or spontaneous miscarriage. In severe cases of iodine deficiency, babies are born with significant and permanent impairment of mental function, hearing, speech, and physical growth, a condition called cretinism.

However, even mild iodine deficiency during pregnancy has been associated with a higher incidence of children with attention-deficit-hyperactive disorder (ADHD) and lower IQs. A meta-analysis of 18 studies found that iodine deficiency lowered mean IQ scores by 13.5 points! So, are women and their children at risk in the United States? Yes! According to the CDC's *Second National Report on Biochemical Indicators of Diet and Nutrition in the U.S. Population* young women (aged 20–39 years) had significantly lower iodine intake compared with other age groups, only slightly above the "insufficient intake" level.

The American Thyroid Association recommends that pregnant women take a prenatal vitamin that provides 150 mcg of iodine every day. Well, many prenatal vitamins don't contain iodine and even if they do, is 150 mcg enough? A 2014 study conducted by Mount Sinai found, after randomly sampling urine for iodine status, that more than one out of two pregnant women in New York City were at risk for iodine deficiency. Still more concerning was that even after supplementing the women with 150 mcg per day of iodine, our current recommendation, more than 20 percent were still at risk for iodine deficiency according to WHO guidelines!

Low levels of iodine may be particularly problematic in women who are deficient in iron. That's because iron forms part of the thyroid peroxidase enzyme, which is necessary for making thyroid hormone. It's a double whammy. The CDC report mentioned above found overall 10.4 percent of women 12 to 49 years of age are deficient in iron (approximately 8 million women), with

Latinas and black women having the highest risk at 12 percent and 16 percent respectively.

Countries once thought to be iodine sufficient, such as the U.S., the United Kingdom, and Australia, are increasingly witnessing iodine insufficiency. This is in no small part due to the dramatic increase in consumption of processed foods. The salt used in U.S. fast foods and roughly 99 percent of processed foods, is non-iodized. Moreover, we've been told to limit our salt intake to reduce the risk of high blood pressure, cardiac disease, and cancer. The "cut back on salt" messages have finally hit home—literally. The place where we have dramatically cut back on salt is at home; one of the few places we can actually use iodized salt. Now our salt shakers are filled with pretty pink Himalayan or kosher salts. Unless the label says the salt is "iodized," you're getting very little iodine. Although salt is one your best sources of daily iodine, a 2007 study found that once salt is opened and exposed to air, up to 40 percent of its iodine is lost after just four weeks.

R℞ RX FROM DR. LOW DOG

Iodine and Radiation

The FDA has approved the use of potassium iodide as a thyroid-blocking agent to reduce the risk of thyroid cancer in radiation emergencies, such as when a nuclear power plant leaks radioactive materials into the atmosphere. The doses are high (16–130 mg per day, depending on age) and should be used only under the direction of a health-care professional.

WHAT TO EAT: Seaweed has highly concentrated levels of highly bioavailable iodine, making it the top food source. Kelp is highest in iodine; dulse, nori, and wakame contain lower amounts. Other food sources include shellfish, fish, cow's milk, and eggs. One teaspoon of iodized salt contains roughly 400 mcg of potassium iodide, but this level may be closer to 240 mcg per teaspoon within 1 to 2 months after opening the package. Because of this loss, the WHO recommends iodization with potassium *iodate* due to its greater stability, particularly in humid, tropical parts of the world.

SIGNS OF DEFICIENCY: The signs of iodine deficiency are the same as for hypoactive thyroid: dry skin, poor memory, slow thinking, fatigue, muscle cramps, weak muscles, intolerance to cold, hoarse voice, puffy eyes, and constipation. And while fibromyalgia is a complex condition, a number of clinicians believe iodine deficiency may play a role in this pain disorder.

Iodine deficiency in school-age children results in learning disability and poor growth. In adults, hypothyroidism with all its attendant signs and symptoms develops. Low iodine intake over months to years can cause the thyroid gland to enlarge, growing bigger and bigger over time in an attempt to extract what little iodine is available. This condition is called a goiter.

RISK FOR DEFICIENCY: Diets that exclude iodized salt, seafood, seaweed, and dairy products often lead to low levels of iodine. A 2014 study by researchers at Boston Medical Center found that vegans are at greater risk for iodine deficiency than are vegetarians or those who eat a mixed diet. The Oxford Vegetarian Study found similar results with vegans in the UK. This may be because their diets don't contain seafood, dairy, or eggs and because their marginal iodine intake is combined with a higher intake of goitrogens: food substances that block the synthesis of thyroid hormones and exacerbate iodine deficiency.

All cruciferous vegetables—including arugula, bok choy, broccoli, Brussels sprouts, cabbage, cauliflower, kale, collard greens, mustard greens, turnips, and watercress are considered goitrogenic—can, theoretically, cause goiter. Cooking decreases their goitrogen activity. Genistein and daidzein, compounds in soybeans, also act as goitrogens and inhibit thyroid hormone synthesis. However, these goitrogens do not have any significant impact on thyroid health unless there is coexisting iodine deficiency. *Bottom line: Eat healthy goitrogenic foods and make sure you are getting enough iodine!*

Another important topic to discuss is the potential adverse effects of endocrine disrupting chemicals (EDCs), compounds that interfere with the body's hormones, on thyroid health. A number of these chemicals have been shown to be triggers for Hashimoto's thyroiditis, the primary cause of hypothyroidism in Western countries. Let me give you two clear examples to help you appreciate just how serious this problem of chemical-induced iodine deficiency is.

First, let's look at bromine, an element in the same family as iodine. Bromine competes with iodine at iodine receptors and it usually wins the game, displacing iodine, which is then excreted by the body. Pesticides, especially those used on strawberries, can contain bromine. Baked goods often contain potassium bromate, while some sodas contain brominated vegetable oils.

Second, the chemicals perchlorate, thiocyanate, nitrate, and phthalates can all inhibit the sodium iodine symporter, the pump that allows iodine to be taken up by the thyroid gland. Perchlorate, in particular, may be a bigger problem than we previously thought. From 2002 to 2006, 21,846 women who were less than 16 weeks pregnant were enrolled into the Controlled Antenatal Thyroid Screening Study from clinics in Cardiff, UK, and Turin, Italy. During this study, the women's urine was collected and tested for iodine and perchlorate. Perchlorate was detectable in *all* the women! What's more, their iodine levels were low. (The median was 72 µg/L, when it should be >150 µg/L.) Women with the highest perchlorate levels had 300 percent greater odds of having babies in the lowest 10 percentile for IQ at three years of age. Perchlorate can also be stored in the mammary glands, potentially decreasing the supply of iodide in breast milk. As seen in this large study, women had both high perchlorate *and* low iodine.

Research has shown that people with type 2 diabetes have lower urinary iodine levels than healthy controls. Because thyroid hormone plays a critical role in the actions of insulin, diabetics need to be sure they are getting adequate iodine.

RX FROM DR. LOW DOG
Iodine for Hypothyroidism

Because the United States has been considered "iodine sufficient" for decades, most physicians don't think to check iodine status when hypothyroidism is suspected or initially diagnosed. It's important for clinicians to have iodine deficiency on their radar. Hypothyroidism due to iodine deficiency is easily treatable with iodine supplementation and does not require thyroid hormone replacement. Having enough iodine not only ensures normal thyroid function, it also prevents the entry of endocrine disruptors and goitrogens into the thyroid gland.

RDA/AI: Men: 150 mcg   Women: 150 mcg

Pregnancy: 220 mcg

Breastfeeding: 290 mcg

DV: 150 mcg

UL: The upper limit for iodine has been set at 1,100 mcg per day for adults. Although iodine is necessary for thyroid hormone synthesis, *too much* can actually trigger hypothyroidism. In genetically susceptible individuals, such as those with a family history of thyroid problems, prolonged intake of more than 1,100 mcg per day of iodine may trigger autoimmune thyroiditis and result in hypothyroidism. People with cystic fibrosis may be particularly sensitive to excessive intake of iodine. Several observational studies have found excessive intake to be associated with an increased risk of thyroid papillary cancer.

SUPPLEMENT CONSIDERATIONS: Look for a multivitamin-mineral supplement that provides 100 percent of the DV for iodine. Supplements typically contain potassium iodide or sodium iodide. The potassium iodide in these products, derived from kelp, is highly bioavailable. However, do not purchase kelp tablets unless the actual amount of iodide is provided on the label. This is *very* important! You could be getting hundreds of times the DV without knowing it.

PARTNER NUTRIENTS: The trace mineral selenium is important for converting thyroxine (T4) to the biologically active thyroid hormone triiodothyronine (T3). Selenium may also slow the activity of autoimmune thyroiditis. Be careful not to take excessive amounts of selenium; 100 mcg per day in a multivitamin-mineral supplement is sufficient.

Deficiencies of vitamin A and iron can further exacerbate iodine deficiency. Vitamin A deficiency has been associated with goiter and decreased uptake of iodine by the thyroid. Iron is necessary for synthesizing thyroid hormones, which is particularly relevant for women and young children who are at greater risk for iron deficiency.

SPECIAL POPULATIONS: Iodine requirements increase during pregnancy and lactation. The Endocrine Society and American Thyroid Association recommend that all women who pregnant or who are trying to get pregnant take a prenatal multivitamin-mineral supplement containing 150 mcg of potassium iodide/iodate daily. Only half of prenatal supplements in the marketplace contain iodine and not all contain the recommended 150 mcg. Women who are breastfeeding should continue taking their prenatal supplement to ensure adequate iodine is passed from her breast milk to her baby.

IRON

Iron is a mineral found in both animal and plant foods, as well as in fortified cereals and breads. According to the WHO, iron deficiency is the most common nutrient deficiency in the world, affecting roughly two billion people. The toll it takes in developing nations is staggering. There, the culprit is a combination of iron-deficient diets and chronic infections from parasites, malaria, and tuberculosis. Iron deficiency during pregnancy increases the risk of death for both mother and baby: Iron deficiency anemia contributes to roughly 20 percent of all maternal deaths worldwide. Low iron levels increase the risk that a baby will be born premature and/or with a low birth weight, and can impair the child's cognitive and behavioral development.

In the United States and other Western countries, iron deficiency among women and children still persists. Iron supplements and multivitamins with iron are common and inexpensive, which is good, but as you'll see, taking too much iron is also dangerous. Read on and you'll understand just how much you need and why.

WHAT IT DOES: Iron is necessary for normal growth and development, plays a key role in DNA synthesis, and is an essential component of hemoglobin, the protein in blood that is responsible for carrying oxygen from the lungs to all the tissues of our body. More than 60 percent of our iron is found in our hemoglobin. It is also present in myoglobin, a protein whose job it is to make sure there is sufficient oxygen available to hard-working muscles. When levels of iron drop, there is not enough to support the normal formation of red blood cells. Fewer red blood cells mean less oxygen going to the tissues, especially the muscles. When you try to exercise, your muscles feel weak and your heart beats faster as it tries to get oxygen to all the tissues that need it, and you end up feeling worse than before you went to the gym. Low levels of iron make it hard to thermoregulate in cold weather. You go for a walk with friends and they all feel fine while you start to shiver and can't get warm as your body tries to both oxygenate tissue and minimize heat loss.

Iron plays a critical role in cellular energy production, the synthesis of DNA, normal growth and development, reproduction, immune function, and the detoxification of certain toxins and drugs. Iron is necessary for proper brain function and poor focus and attention are common in kids and adults with low iron. A 2010 meta-analysis in the *Nutrition Journal* that included 14 randomized controlled trials of children over the age of six, adolescents, and adult women who had iron deficiency anemia found that iron supplementation improved attention, concentration, and IQ. I have to wonder if some of these children and teenagers taking psychostimulant medications for ADHD have been thoroughly evaluated for nutritional deficiencies, including iron.

Another condition that may result from iron deficiency is restless leg syndrome (RLS), a neurological condition that causes an uncomfortable creepy-crawling sensation in the legs and a strong urge to move them to reduce the feeling of aching or tingling. The symptoms are most common at night. Roughly 1 in 20 people under the age of 65 and 1 in 10 people over the age of 65 have RLS. Iron deficiency is associated with RLS and even those who have normal serum iron levels may have low levels of iron in their brain tissue. Studies repeatedly show that iron supplements can improve symptoms but it's not currently known how low iron concentration in the brain contributes to RLS. One hypothesis is that low levels of iron alter the activity of an iron-dependent enzyme (tyrosine hydroxylase) making it hard for the body to synthesize dopamine, a neurotransmitter that may be involved in RLS.

Iron deficiency increases the intestinal absorption of lead in humans and animals and may increase the risk of lead poisoning in children.

WHAT TO EAT: There are two forms of iron found in food, heme and non-heme. Meat contains both forms, while plants and fortified foods contain only non-heme iron. We absorb roughly 18 percent of heme iron, compared to about 10 percent of the non-heme iron in plants, which is less bioavailable. Phytic acid, a compound found in beans, rice, and grains, binds to non-heme iron, further reducing its absorption, as does soy protein. So, while soybeans, black beans, lentils, mung beans, and split peas are high in iron, the amount absorbed is low, generally less than 2 percent. However, you can increase the absorption of non-heme iron be eating your legumes with vitamin C. Here in the Southwest, many people cook their black beans with chile (chili) peppers, a great source of vitamin C. Meat, shellfish (such as clams and oysters), nuts, dried fruits, and fortified foods are also good sources of iron. And for the record, Popeye was right! No wonder he was able to pack such a wallop after downing a can of cooked spinach: Cooking spinach increases the bioavailability of its iron. And cooking your food in a cast-iron skillet can also increase the iron in your food.

Studies show that the iron content of 3 ounces of meat spaghetti sauce increased from 0.61 mg to 5.77 mg and scrambled eggs from 1.49 mg to 4.76 mg when these foods were cooked in a cast-iron skillet. As someone who grew up dreading the chore of washing the evening dishes because it meant cleaning my mother's cast-iron skillet, I must say I have newfound appreciation!

SIGNS OF DEFICIENCY: Fatigue, muscle weakness with exertion, rapid heart rate, heart palpitations, and inability to maintain body warmth upon exposure to cold, are all signs of iron deficiency. Spoon-shaped, brittle nails, loss of taste and sore tongue, are signs of more severe iron deficiency anemia.

RISK FOR DEFICIENCY: According to the CDC's *Second National Report on Biochemical Indicators of Diet and Nutrition in the U.S. Population*, roughly 7 percent of children aged one to five are iron deficient, though the numbers are higher for Mexican-American children at 12 percent. In the U.S., approximately 10 percent of women between 12 and 49 years of age have iron deficiency, but looking more closely at ethnicity and race, roughly 12 percent of Latina women and 16 percent of black women are deficient.

Iron demands increase dramatically as pregnancy advances. According to a 2011 review in the *American Journal of Clinical Nutrition* among pregnant women, depleted iron stores are more common in Mexican-American (23.6 percent) and non-Hispanic black women (29.6 percent) than in non-Hispanic white women (13.9 percent). This is very concerning since studies consistently show that the incidence of having a premature birth and/or a low-birth-weight baby is far more prevalent for black women. While we are making strides for reducing iron deficiency in the U.S., it is clear we still have a long way to go.

Iron deficiency can result from low dietary intake, poor iron absorption, or excessive and/or prolonged blood loss. Women lose iron through menstruation—typically 15 to 20 mg each month—so they need to eat plenty of iron-rich foods throughout the month and consider taking multivitamin-mineral with iron. If you are a healthy person who donates blood (thank you!), you probably also need an iron supplement. One clinical trial that enrolled people who had donated blood found that without iron supplementation, two-thirds of the donors had not recovered the iron they lost, even after 24 weeks. Blood loss from any cause may impact your iron stores.

Keep in mind that chronic blood loss may not be readily apparent. I had a close friend who was 54 years old, past the age where she was losing blood regularly due to menstruation, yet she'd had iron deficiency anemia for about two years. Finally, her doctor recommended that she have a colonoscopy. She was diagnosed with colon cancer. The point I'm trying to make is that it's important to know *why* someone has iron deficiency anemia and not just assume that taking iron supplements will fix the problem.

In many cases, however, the reasons for iron deficiency are far more obvious. Here's a fairly common scenario I've experienced: A mother of two or three young children would come to see me, saying that she felt exhausted, was cold, had no energy, couldn't focus, and felt tired after exercising. I would order some laboratory tests and almost always, the results showed the woman had iron deficiency anemia. Repeated pregnancies, breastfeeding and a poor diet often leave women with low levels of iron. The other common reason for iron deficiency is heavy menstrual periods, particularly in women with uterine fibroids or during the menopausal years.

Gastric bypass (bariatric) surgery can increase the risk of iron deficiency by impairing absorption. Other conditions that might require iron supplementation include kidney failure, heart failure, Crohn's disease, and ulcerative colitis.

RDA/AI: Men: 8 mg   Women: 19–50: 18 mg
         After 50: 8 mg
         Pregnancy: 27 mg
         Breastfeeding: 9 mg

RDA/AI FOR VEGETARIANS: Men: 14 mg Women 19–50:
                 33 mg
                 After 50: 14 mg

Note: The RDA for vegetarians is 1.8 times higher than for people who eat a mixed diet that includes meat.

DV: 18 mg

UL: 45 mg. The tolerable upper intake limit does not apply to those being treated for iron deficiency anemia.

WARNING!
Be Careful of Iron Supplements Around Children!

Keep iron supplements out of the reach of children. The FDA mandates that all iron supplements bear the following on their label: "WARNING! Accidental overdose of iron-containing products is a leading cause of fatal poisoning in children under 6. Keep this product out of reach of children. In case of accidental overdose, call a doctor or poison control center immediately." With increasing numbers of iron-containing, candy-like chewable vitamins, it's more important than ever to keep all vitamins out of the reach of children to prevent poisoning.

SUPPLEMENT CONSIDERATIONS: A multivitamin containing the DV of iron is a good idea if you are a menstruating, pregnant, or breastfeeding woman. Children also benefit from a basic multivitamin that provides 50 to 100 percent of the DV of iron for their age. People who are not at risk of iron deficiency (teenage boys, adult men, women with very infrequent menstrual cycles, and postmenopausal women) should *not* take multivitamin-mineral supplements that contain iron or iron supplements unless instructed to do so by their health-care provider. Studies show that men are getting too much iron!

The amount of iron absorbed decreases as the amount ingested increases, which is why it is generally recommended that adults take 50 to 60 mg of elemental iron *twice* a day if they have been diagnosed with iron deficiency anemia.

Iron comes in a variety of forms in dietary supplements. Ferrous fumarate contains the most elemental iron, but both it and ferrous sulfate tend to be the most constipating, nausea-inducing forms. They'll certainly correct the anemia, but many people, especially pregnant women, find them hard on the stomach. Chelated forms of iron are better tolerated, so they can be a good choice even though you may have to take more tablets to get the amount of iron you need. Look for iron bisglycinate, ferrous bisglycinate, or iron glycinate on the label. Food-based iron products are also available and are probably the best tolerated of all the forms.

Do not take iron supplements at the same time you take your calcium supplements or within a couple hours of drinking coffee, tea, or cow's milk as these substances all decrease the absorption of iron.

PARTNER NUTRIENTS: Vitamin C increases iron absorption, especially from non-heme (plant) sources. Vitamin A helps iron partner with hemoglobin, the protein that allows blood cells to carry oxygen throughout the body. Riboflavin improves iron absorption and utilization. Copper is needed to transport iron to the bone marrow to make red blood cells. When copper is low, iron accumulates in the liver. A basic multivitamin-mineral product generally provides adequate amounts of vitamin A, riboflavin, and copper. Make sure you take additional zinc if taking

WARNING!
Avoid Excess Iron

Although iron is an essential mineral, it can be toxic when taken in excess because the body has no easy way of getting rid of it except through bleeding. It accumulates in our organs and wreaks havoc. It can cause scarring and cirrhosis of the liver. Excess iron in the pancreas leads to diabetes—and in the heart it leads to heart failure. Excess iron may also be dangerous to the brain, increasing the risk for neurodegenerative disease. Too much iron is particularly problematic for those that have a genetic disorder called hemochromatosis, which causes iron to be absorbed and stored at much higher rates. Affecting 1 in 200 individuals of northern European descent, hemochromatosis is one of the most common genetic disorders in the United States. One of the primary treatments is phlebotomy, or essentially, donating blood. Roughly a pint of blood is removed once a week until iron levels return to normal. This procedure it is repeated every two to four months to ensure that the levels don't build up again. *Bottom line: If you are not a young child, menstruating or pregnant/breastfeeding woman, do not take supplemental iron unless instructed to by your health-care provider.* So, even though iron is often effective for treating RLS, make sure you discuss using it with your health-care provider first, so your iron levels can be monitored.

high-dose iron supplements for the treatment of iron deficiency anemia, as it can reduce the absorption of zinc. Take iron and zinc supplements with food for maximum absorption.

SPECIAL POPULATIONS: During pregnancy the body dramatically increases production of red blood cells to meet the needs of both the mother and the baby growing inside her. More red blood cells require more iron and hemoglobin. If you are pregnant, your physician or midwife will check your iron levels early in the pregnancy and again before you enter your third trimester. If you need additional iron, you will be given supplements. Otherwise, look for a good prenatal multivitamin-mineral supplement that provides the RDA of iron for pregnant women.

Menstruating women need a constant supply of iron to counter the monthly loss from menstruation. Because iron from plants is less efficiently absorbed than that from animals, the Food and Nutrition Board recommends that the RDA for vegetarians and vegans be 1.8 times the standard RDA for iron. People who engage in regular intense exercise may need up to 30 percent more iron than the RDA.

MAGNESIUM

Government surveys show that roughly 50 percent of us don't get the RDA for magnesium in our diet—and many of us take medications, such as diuretics and proton pump inhibitors, which can wipe out the magnesium we are getting. You'd think we would be hearing more about this in the news given all the really important jobs magnesium performs in our body.

Chronically low levels of magnesium have been linked to diabetes, high blood pressure, heart disease, sudden cardiac death, migraines, menstrual cramps, depression, osteoporosis, and asthma. Magnesium is involved in the workings of more than 300 enzyme systems in the body. Without magnesium, these enzymes can't perform their duties. Magnesium is the fourth most abundant mineral in our body, and the adult skeleton is its primary storage depot, holding over 60 percent of the body's magnesium reserves. Another 30 percent or so of our magnesium is found in our muscles and soft tissue, 6 to 7 percent is found inside of our cells, and the remaining 1 percent exists in the blood and extracellular fluid.

WHAT IT DOES: Magnesium is involved in the metabolism of carbohydrates and fats and the production of DNA, RNA, and other proteins. It is also actively involved with cell signaling, nerve impulses, muscle contractions, and maintaining a normal heart rhythm. Magnesium is required for the synthesis of glutathione, one of our body's most powerful antioxidant and detoxifying agents.

Magnesium is extremely important for cardiovascular health. A 2013 meta-analysis published in the *American Journal of Clinical Nutrition* that included 16 studies and more than 313,000 participants found higher blood levels of magnesium were associated with a 30 percent lower risk of cardiovascular disease. It relaxes blood vessels, lowering blood pressure. A comprehensive review of 44 human studies published in the journal *Magnesium Research* in 2013 found that magnesium supplementation (230–460 mg per day) increased the effectiveness of blood pressure medications in people with stage one hypertension (blood pressures ranging from 140/90 to 159/99). It didn't matter what type of medication was used—a little magnesium made them all work better. Since many of the medications that are used to treat hypertension actually deplete magnesium, supplementing makes sense.

During pregnancy, usually after 20 weeks' gestation, some women develop preeclampsia, a condition characterized by high blood pressure, protein in the urine, and swelling of the legs. Preeclampsia affects up to 8 percent of pregnancies, and if left untreated, blood pressure rises to dangerous levels and seizures can develop—a condition called eclampsia. As you can imagine, eclampsia is very dangerous for both the mother and baby. While calcium supplementation reduces the risk of preeclampsia it is magnesium that is used to treat preeclampsia and eclampsia. A 2010 review of seven studies by the Cochrane Group concluded that magnesium is the drug of choice for women with eclampsia, reducing the risk of seizures and maternal death, and improving the health of the newborn.

Magnesium is very important for reducing the risk of heart arrhythmias. Sudden cardiac death occurs when the heart stops beating suddenly and unexpectedly, accounting for more than 50 percent of all cardiovascular deaths. When Harvard researchers evaluated more than 88,000 women taking part in the Nurses' Health Study, they found that those with the highest blood magnesium levels had roughly a 77 percent lower risk of dying from sudden cardiac death! The Framingham Offspring Study found similar results: Those with low serum magnesium levels (≤ 1.77 mg/dL) had a 50 percent greater risk for atrial fibrillation when compared to those with the highest levels (≥ 1.99 mg/dL).

Magnesium may also protect us from stroke by making our platelets less likely to form blood clots. (Blood clots can stick to the inside walls of arteries and reduce or cut off blood flow, causing a stroke.) In the Japan Collaborative Cohort Study, dietary magnesium intake was recorded for 58,615 healthy Japanese aged 40 to 79. During the 14.7-year follow-up, researchers found that the higher the magnesium intake, the lower a man's risk of dying from stroke and the lower a woman's risk of dying from stroke, heart failure, and coronary artery disease.

Magnesium helps maintain a healthy blood sugar, preventing diabetes and improving the health of those with the disease. This is worth noting, because according to the CDC, if current trends continue, one in three American adults will have diabetes by 2050. That is a shocking statistic! Magnesium may be one piece of this complex puzzle of dramatic increases in type 2 diabetes. A 2011 review of 13 studies and more than 530,000 people published in *Diabetes Care*, the journal of the American Diabetes Association, found that those with the highest magnesium intake had a 22 percent lower risk for developing type 2 diabetes, especially if they were overweight or obese.

When blood sugars rise, magnesium is excreted in the urine. Up to one-third of people with diabetes are deficient in magnesium, further complicating their ability to maintain good blood sugar control: a vicious cycle. A meta-analysis by researchers at Brigham and Women's Hospital and Harvard Medical School found that oral magnesium supplementation (median dose was 360 mg per day) for 4 to 16 weeks in people with type 2 diabetes significantly lowered fasting blood glucose levels and increased HDL cholesterol (the good kind of cholesterol) when compared to placebo groups.

Metabolic syndrome is the name given to a group of risk factors that increase your likelihood of developing heart disease, stroke, and type 2 diabetes. Given what we've just discussed, it makes sense that magnesium should help protect us from this condition. And that's just what the research shows! People with low serum magnesium levels are up to seven times more likely to develop metabolic syndrome than are those with normal levels. This protective effect may be due in part to the fact that higher intakes of magnesium lower C-reactive protein, an indicator of inflammation in the body. It is now believed that chronic low-grade inflammation is a major driver of heart disease, diabetes, osteoporosis, cancer, and even depression.

Magnesium is important for bone health, in part because of its role in the regulation and metabolism of calcium and vitamin D, but also because it is one of the key minerals that make up our bones. As magnesium levels in bone decrease, bones become more brittle. A 2014 meta-analysis of seven studies published in the journal *Biological Trace Mineral Research* found that low serum magnesium is a risk factor for postmenopausal osteoporosis. Studies in both elder men and women have shown that higher intakes of magnesium are positively associated with better bone density of the hip and spine.

Magnesium is a calming mineral that nourishes the nervous system and helps ease anxiety, irritability, and depression. Low levels of magnesium reduce serotonin levels, a neurotransmitter associated with a healthy mood. I encourage anyone dealing with depression or anxiety to make sure they are getting plenty of magnesium in their diet and to consider additional supplementation. There is a small body of research suggesting that when magnesium levels are low, symptoms of ADHD may be exacerbated. Because many children and adolescents do not meet the RDA for magnesium, for them, a multivitamin or magnesium supplement that provides 75 to 150 mg of magnesium per day might be in order.

People with migraines often have low brain levels of serotonin and magnesium. I see a connection here! Research shows that taking 400 to 600 mg of magnesium per day reduces the number and severity of migraines in adults. One study in children found supplementing with 9 mg of magnesium per kilogram (2.2 pounds) of body weight per day reduced the frequency of migraines. The Canadian Headache Society gives magnesium citrate a strong recommendation for the prevention of migraines. The American Academy of Neurology and the American Headache Society give magnesium a level B recommendation, the same level as for the pain relievers, ibuprofen and naproxen. As someone with migraines, I can tell you magnesium has made a huge difference in my own life. On a few occasions, I've forgotten to bring my magnesium while traveling. I have no problem for two or three days and then wham! A migraine! When it comes to magnesium, just like my American Express card, I never leave home without it.

Women who suffer from monthly menstrual cramps may find that magnesium will bring some relief. A 2009 review in *American Family Physician*, the official journal of the American Academy of Family Practice, found promising evidence that magnesium can help relieve symptoms of dysmenorrhea and alleviate leg cramps in women who are pregnant. One study found that taking 500 mg per day starting at the onset of menstruation reduced cramping pain. And if you feel anxious and irritable around your menstrual cycle, it might interest you to know that when women took 200 mg of magnesium and 50 mg of vitamin B6 every day, they experienced a significant improvement in their mood, as well as reductions in breast tenderness, menstrual weight gain, and pain. Taking magnesium at bedtime can help relax your muscles, prevent nasty middle-of-the-night leg cramps, and promote a restful sleep.

And finally, magnesium plays an important role in asthma. A 2014 review by the Cochrane Group found that a single intravenous dose of magnesium administered in the emergency room improved lung function and reduced hospital admissions in those patients who did not respond well to other interventions.

Whew! Now can you see why I want to get the word out about this marvelous mineral and its benefits?

WHAT TO EAT: Magnesium is found in both plant and animal foods. Cooked spinach, black beans, pumpkin seeds, almonds, cashews, soy milk, peanut butter, avocados, whole wheat bread, brown rice, yogurt, salmon, and milk are all good sources of magnesium. Of course, my favorite source of magnesium would have to be dark chocolate! Also, to ensure you get all the magnesium you need, make certain that your diet contains adequate amounts of protein. When protein intake is less than 30 grams per day (equivalent to 3 ounces of red meat or 1 cup of cooked beans), magnesium absorption falls.

SIGNS OF DEFICIENCY: People with magnesium deficiency may have insulin resistance, menstrual cramps, leg cramps, migraines, fatigue, anxiety and mild elevations in blood pressure. In more severe cases of deficiency, seizures, tingling and numbness in the arms and legs, personality changes, and coronary spasms can occur

RISK FOR DEFICIENCY: Alcoholism, diabetes, and gastrointestinal diseases, such as Crohn's disease (which causes malabsorption of many nutrients), can all cause magnesium depletion. Low magnesium levels often occur in older people due to decreased absorption in the GI tract.

Large amounts of fiber can impair magnesium absorption. Take your fiber supplement or high-fiber cereal in the morning and your magnesium at night. High calcium intake (>2,500 mg/day) in combination with a high-sodium diet enhances magnesium excretion. Just one more reason not to overdo the calcium supplements and to watch the salt!

Women: Be aware that it is possible that low levels of magnesium increase a woman's risk for both blood clots and strokes if she is taking estrogen in her oral contraceptive or hormone therapy during menopause. The risk is greater in women who are low in magnesium when they start taking estrogen. Interestingly, many women complain that oral contraceptives trigger headaches—and low levels of magnesium are associated with migraines. I recommend that any woman taking estrogen should ensure that she is getting adequate magnesium to protect her bones, brain, and cardiovascular system.

RDA/AI: Men: 420 mg   Women: 320 mg
Pregnancy: 350 mg
Breastfeeding: 320 mg

DV: 400 mg

UL: 350 mg (for supplements only). *Note:* This upper limit only applies to magnesium supplements, not food. Magnesium is widely used as a laxative for the treatment of constipation. An upper limit of 350 mg has been set because higher doses of supplements are likely to cause diarrhea. Also, higher doses are not safe in someone who has very poor kidney function.

SUPPLEMENT CONSIDERATIONS: Most of us would benefit from taking 200 to 300 mg of magnesium per day as a supplement. If you are dealing with migraines or taking medications that deplete magnesium, you might need to take 400 to 600 mg per day. Because magnesium can interfere with a number of medications and because it helps our muscles relax, its best to take at bedtime.

Magnesium supplements are available in a variety of forms. Magnesium oxide is the least expensive and also the most likely to cause intestinal cramping and diarrhea. To avoid those problems, look for chelated magnesium, magnesium malate, magnesium glycinate, or magnesium bisglycinate. These forms are gentler on the stomach, less likely to cause diarrhea, and easily absorbed. Magnesium citrate is a middle-of-the-road choice, good for those who could benefit from magnesium and a mild laxative.

Magnesium can be absorbed through the skin to some degree. Bathing with Epsom salts (magnesium sulfate) or using magnesium gel or lotion topically can be helpful for relaxing muscles and easing leg cramps.

WARNING!
Avoid Magnesium Supplements If You Have Poor Kidney Function

Since poor kidney function makes it much more difficult to excrete excess magnesium, people with serious kidney disease should only take magnesium supplements under the supervision of their health-care provider.

PARTNER NUTRIENTS: Magnesium, calcium and vitamin D all work together in the body. Make sure you are getting adequate amounts of all of them on a regular basis. At doses of more than 250 mg, magnesium may interfere with absorption of trace minerals and compete with calcium for absorption, so take high doses of magnesium several hours apart from your multivitamin and calcium.

SPECIAL POPULATIONS: Everyone, young and old, with healthy kidneys should increase his or her dietary intake of magnesium.

POTASSIUM

Potassium is critically important to our health. Low levels in the body increase our risk for high blood pressure, heart disease, stroke, infertility, and possibly even cancer. Having too little or too much is dangerous (see box). I cannot stress how important it is to ensure that you are getting adequate amounts of potassium *in your diet*.

WARNING!
Get Your Potassium Through Healthy Eating!

The recommended daily intake for potassium is 4,700 mg, but since high-dose potassium supplementation requires close monitoring, you will not find commercial dietary supplements that contain more than 99 mg of elemental potassium per serving. That's only 3% of the DV per tablet. That means you would have to take 47 potassium pills in one day to meet the RDA! The only way to get the potassium you need is by eating plenty of potassium-rich foods. Here are a few of the best sources: One baked potato with skin has about 920 milligrams of potassium, one sweet potato contains around 700 mg, 2 ounces of tomato paste provide 660 mg, 1 cup of plain yogurt 580 mg, 3 ounces of tuna or 1/2 cup of cooked soybeans provides 500 mg, 1 cup of orange juice has 500 mg, one medium banana has 400 mg, while 1 cup of skim milk contains 382 mg (whole milk has a little less). So, load up!

SELENIUM

Selenium is a naturally occurring substance widely distributed in the earth's crust and sedimentary rock, and found in small amounts in our water, soil, and food. The name is derived from *selene*, named for the Greek goddess of the moon, surely a reference to the fact that the electrical conductivity of selenium increases as much as a thousandfold when taken from pure darkness into bright sunlight. In fact, selenium is often used in the manufacture of light meters and solar cells. Human beings need only trace amounts to carry out a number of metabolic and antioxidant processes. Selenium is an essential nutrient in human health but can be toxic in excess.

WHAT IT DOES: Selenium is an essential trace element necessary for the proper function of two vitally important enzymes, glutathione peroxidase and thioredoxin reductase. These enzymes act as potent antioxidants in our body, protecting our DNA from damage. Selenium is also involved in the production of immune T-cells, which are necessary for destroying cells that have been infected with viruses or bacteria or have become cancerous. Selenium deficiency increases our risk for viral infections, while supplementation might protect people infected with the hepatitis B or C virus from developing liver cancer. Low levels of selenium are thought to be associated with an increased risk for colorectal, stomach, lung, and prostate cancer. However, a large study called the SELECT trial, which gave men 200 mcg per day of selenium, failed to find any reduction in the risk for prostate, lung, or colorectal cancer. The reason for the discrepancy in studies is not clear.

Selenium is needed to convert the thyroid hormone thyroxine (T4) to the biologically active triiodothyronine (T3). Maintaining the right ratio between these two thyroid hormones is important, and when T3 levels are low, it can cause hypothyroid symptoms. Selenium may be particularly important for those who have autoimmune thyroid disorders.

The most common cause of hypothyroidism in Western countries is Hashimoto's thyroiditis, and selenium shows promise as a treatment. We know that selenium helps protect the thyroid gland from oxidative damage (cellular imbalances that lead to

DNA damage and even the growth of cancer cells). We also know it lowers thyroid-specific antibody levels, which happens when your body's immune cells begin to attack your thyroid gland. Studies show that taking 200 mcg per day of selenium in combination with levothyroxine (a thyroid medication) significantly reduces thyroid peroxidase antibodies by up to 30 percent more than placebo in adults with Hashimoto's thyroiditis after 3 to 12 months of treatment. If you are being treated for Hashimoto's thyroiditis, make sure you talk to your health-care practitioner about taking selenium!

During pregnancy, to prevent the immune system's attacking the fetus as something "foreign," a woman's immune system is suppressed to protect her child. After the baby is born, the immune system rebounds rapidly and sometimes there is a worsening of autoimmune conditions, including thyroiditis. Interestingly, a 2013 review of studies by the international Cochrane Group found that selenium supplementation during pregnancy decreases the incidence of moderate to severe postpartum thyroiditis. This finding is important given that 20 to 40 percent of women who develop postpartum thyroiditis will go on to have permanent hypothyroidism.

There is an important relationship between selenium and iodine in our body. While it has been thought that the United States was iodine sufficient, as I discussed in the "Iodine" section (see page XXX), a number of us may be at risk for deficiency. I point this out because if you take selenium supplements *and* you are iodine deficient, it can actually *worsen* hypothyroidism. Taking a multivitamin-mineral supplement that gives you the DV of both these crucial minerals is a wise approach.

Selenium is important for the reproductive health of both men and women. Selenium, like zinc, is necessary for the production of testosterone and development of sperm. Low levels are associated with a decrease in male fertility. Low selenium levels also appear to be associated with first trimester and/or recurrent miscarriages.

Finally, selenium may offer some protection against some of the toxic effects of heavy metals such as cadmium, silver, and mercury in seafood.

WHAT TO EAT: Brazil nuts and beef kidney are two of the most absorbable forms of selenium. Shrimp, crabmeat, salmon, pork, chicken, beef, whole grains, garlic, onions and leeks are also good sources.

Agricultural practices and geographical differences can have a significant impact on the selenium content of both food crops and in animals consumed for meat. Although selenium occurs in some soils, industrial farming can deplete it. Selenium is also lost during processing and boiling. We must consider all of these factors when evaluating the "average" selenium content of foods.

SIGNS OF DEFICIENCY: Signs of deficiency can include muscular weakness and pain. In more severe cases, selenium deficiency can cause a very specific form of heart disease in women and children known as Keshan disease. Over time, the deficiency leads to an enlargement of the heart, or cardiomyopathy, and eventually, heart failure. Keshan disease has been noted primarily in a region of China where the soil is very deficient in selenium. Selenium supplementation can prevent Keshan disease from developing, but it can't reverse the heart damage once it has occurred. Another disease potentially related to selenium is Kashin-Beck disease, a type of arthritis that typically affects children in parts of northern China and Siberia. Joint deformities can be significant, and in severe forms, dwarfism can occur. It is thought that selenium deficiency is the cause or a contributing factor in Kashin-Beck disease.

RISK FOR DEFICIENCY: People with HIV, who are pregnant, chronically ill, on kidney dialysis, receiving prolonged intravenous feedings, or who have thyroid disease may be at risk for selenium deficiency.

RDA/AI: Men: 55 mcg   Women: 55 mcg
Pregnancy: 60 mcg
Breastfeeding: 70 mcg

DV: 70 mcg

UL: 400 mcg. Although the upper limit has been set at 400 mcg per day, I never recommend taking more than 200 mcg per day without monitoring blood levels. In those with adequate levels of selenium, taking too much selenium in supplements can be dangerous. A long-term study found that men taking 200 mcg per day for an average of five and a half years had an increased risk of aggressive prostate cancer if their *baseline* selenium was high. As most people do not know what their selenium levels are, it is best to stick with doses under 100 mcg per day.

SUPPLEMENT CONSIDERATIONS: Look for products that contain selenomethionine or yeast-bound selenium. In general, taking a multivitamin-mineral supplement that provides 100 percent of the DV (70 mcg) should be adequate. If I am recommending 200 mcg per day for longer than a few months, I monitor blood levels of selenium to ensure against excessive accumulation or oversupplementing.

PARTNER NUTRIENTS: Selenium partners with copper, iron, and zinc to form antioxidant enzymes. Selenium deficiency combined with iodine deficiency can increase the risk for hypothyroidism.

Selenium requires activated B6 (P5P) for absorption. Always take selenium as part of a multivitamin-mineral supplement.

SPECIAL POPULATIONS: See safety warnings under "Risk for deficiency," page XXX).

ZINC

. . . .

Zinc is the second most abundant trace mineral in the body. (Iron is the first.) Because our body doesn't have an effective way to store zinc, it must be replaced regularly in the diet. Zinc was found to be an essential mineral in human beings in 1961. Since then, it has become clear that mild forms of zinc deficiency are present across the globe, affecting up to one-quarter of the world's population. Low zinc levels can make us more vulnerable to infection, which is particularly true in Africa, the eastern Mediterranean, and Southeast Asia, where zinc deficiency is associated with diarrheal diseases, pneumonia, and malaria. The World Health Organization estimates that marginal zinc status results in the deaths of more than 780,000 children under the age of five every year from these three conditions. Zinc supplements have been shown to lessen the duration and frequency of diarrheal episodes, as well as reduce the severity of pneumonia in malnourished children, saving the lives of many in developing nations. The true health burden of marginal deficiency is really unknown, however, as there are no reliable and easy tests to determine zinc levels currently available.

WHAT IT DOES: Zinc has many roles to play in the body. It is involved in numerous enzymatic reactions, including those that are necessary for the expression of hundreds of our genes. Remember, genes are sets of instructions found in our DNA within the nucleus of our cells. And within this nucleus, you'll find an abundance of zinc, where it assists in the replication, transcription, and repair of our DNA. Because zinc affects DNA, a woman's need for zinc is increased during pregnancy. Maternal zinc deficiency can cause abnormal growth and development in the baby. Having adequate levels of zinc during pregnancy has been shown to reduce the incidence of premature birth by up to 14 percent in low-income women.. Zinc continues to be vitally important for growth, weight gain, and the neurological development during infancy and childhood.

Men have a higher daily requirement for zinc because it is used in the production of testosterone, making it an important nutrient for male sexual maturation and reproduction. Zinc concentrations are very high in the prostate gland, testes, and in sperm. Deficiency of this important trace mineral might contribute to lower testosterone levels and infertility in men. Some small studies have found that zinc supplementation can improve sperm count and enhance fertility.

Zinc plays a vital role in our immune response. We need zinc to activate T-lymphocytes, the immune cells responsible for destroying cells that have been infected with viruses or bacteria, or that have become cancerous. Marginal zinc deficiency can also diminish the activity of other important immune cells, such as macrophages, neutrophils, and natural killer cells. You can easily see why so many vulnerable children, deficient in zinc, die from infection in poor countries.

While most people reach for the vitamin C when they get a cold, there is actually better evidence for zinc. A review by the international Cochrane Group concluded that zinc lozenges are beneficial in reducing the duration and severity of the common cold in healthy people when taken within 24 hours of the onset of symptoms. Another study found that children taking a basic zinc supplement for at least five months had fewer colds, missed less school, and were less likely to be prescribed antibiotics. I encourage you to keep some zinc lozenges on hand. I travel with a few in my purse in case I start coming down with a cold.

Our body needs zinc, along with vitamin C and other nutrients, to heal wounds. Zinc activates the proteins needed to synthesize collagen, while also activating collagenase, an enzyme that allows your cells to reassemble collagen during wound healing. Topically applied zinc preparations enhance the healing of hard-to-mend wounds, such as chronic leg ulcers and bedsores. And most mothers are familiar with the use of zinc oxide paste for treating diaper rash! Collagen is an important component of tendons, cartilage, and bone. And this is where the vast majority of zinc is stored: in our muscles, connective tissues, and bone.

Speaking of bones, zinc levels are often low in people with osteoporosis. A 2014 study published in the journal of *Clinical Interventions in Aging* found that zinc levels were very low in the hip bones of people who had suffered a fracture. Zinc is involved in the mineralization of bone, which increases its strength, making it less likely to break, so low zinc may have contributed to those fractures. A growing body of evidence suggests that osteoporosis may be driven, in part, by chronic low-grade inflammation in the body. Low levels of zinc lead to higher levels of inflammatory compounds in our body; thus, zinc may inhibit this inflammatory-driven loss of bone mineral density. Some research suggests that taking zinc in combination with copper, manganese, and calcium may protect against postmenopausal bone loss.

Zinc is a structural component of numerous antioxidant enzymes, including superoxide dismutase, one of our body's most potent antioxidants and also a powerful anti-inflammatory. When zinc levels are low, the synthesis of these enzymes is impaired and our body experiences greater oxidative stress, which can damage

DNA and contribute to the progression of chronic disease. One classic example is diabetes.

People with diabetes have significantly higher levels of DNA damage than do healthy age-matched controls, which may help explain their increased risk for eye, kidney, and cardiovascular disease. Zinc is necessary for insulin synthesis and storage. In the pancreas, zinc helps protect the beta cells that are responsible for producing insulin. Zinc also makes the body's cells more receptive to insulin, reducing the risk of insulin resistance. All of this helps to maintain healthy, stable blood sugar. Studies have shown that people with type 1 and type 2 diabetes have poor zinc absorption and greater excretion of zinc in their urine. (See "Chromium" on page XXX for more information about diabetes.) Those with more severe diabetes have been shown to have significantly lower levels of serum zinc; it's a vicious cycle.

Zinc is important for our eyesight, hearing, taste, and sense of smell. It is needed to produce retinol-binding protein, which delivers vitamin A to the retina where it helps us see in dim light. In other words, zinc works together with vitamin A to protect our vision, particularly our night vision. It is also important for protecting our eyes as we age.

The Age-Related Eye Disease Study (AREDS) was a randomized, placebo-controlled trial that included more than 3,500 people. It was designed to see whether high doses of antioxidants (500 mg of vitamin C, 400 IU of vitamin E, and 25,000 IU of beta-carotene) with or without zinc (80 mg as zinc oxide) would slow the progression of age-related macular degeneration (AMD), a leading cause of blindness. After roughly six years, it was shown that supplementation with antioxidants plus zinc (but not antioxidants alone) significantly reduced the risk of developing advanced AMD and loss of vision. Eighty milligrams far exceeds the upper limit for zinc, so it was wonderful when the AREDS 2 trial found that antioxidants plus just 25 mg of zinc offered the same protection as the higher dose.

Zinc is necessary for your sense of smell, which accounts for about 80 percent of your sense of taste! It is also important for the health of your mouth; one sign of zinc deficiency is red, swollen, and tender gums that often bleed after brushing. Studies suggest that zinc supplements can reduce recurrent canker sores and also protect the cells that line the mouth in those undergoing chemotherapy and/or radiation. Changes in taste are relatively common for those undergoing cancer treatment. Several studies have shown that zinc supplements can prevent radiation-induced taste changes when taken at the beginning of treatment and continued through one month after treatment is completed.

Zinc may offer some protection against depression. Recurrent major depression has been associated with decreased blood zinc concentrations, which may be further diminished by antidepressant medication. A 2012 systemic review of four randomized controlled trials published in the *Journal of Affective Disorders* suggested that zinc supplementation might be beneficial when combined with conventional antidepressant medications.

WHAT TO EAT: While oysters win for having the highest concentration of zinc, red meat and chicken are the primary sources of zinc in the American diet. Zinc from these foods is also among the best absorbed. That's because animal proteins, including those in seafood, enhance zinc absorption. Vegetarians may need 50 percent more zinc than those with mixed diets, as the zinc in plants is more difficult to absorb due to the presence of phytic acid (see discussion under "Iron," page XXX).

SIGNS OF DEFICIENCY: Low zinc can cause an altered sense of taste or smell, impotence in men, weight loss, hair loss, mental fatigue, diarrhea, slow healing of wounds, and poor night vision. Unfortunately, most of these signs and symptoms are nonspecific—they could be caused by any number of conditions and not just zinc deficiency. And since there is no really good laboratory test to determine zinc levels, clinicians have to use their best judgment to determine whether a patient is zinc deficient.

RISK FOR DEFICIENCY: Children, adolescents, pregnant and breastfeeding women, vegetarians and vegans are all at risk for zinc deficiency. Deficiency is also more likely in those who've had weight-loss surgery, drink more than two servings per day of alcohol, or have sickle cell anemia, Crohn's disease, ulcerative colitis, rheumatoid arthritis, kidney disease, liver disease, diabetes, or asthma. That's quite a list.

RDA: Men: 11 mg

Women: 8 mg
Pregnancy: 11 mg
Breastfeeding: 12 mg

DV: 15 mg

UL: 40 mg .It is important not to exceed the upper limit for zinc for more than just a short period of time, such as in the case of using zinc lozenges for a cold. Intakes of 60 mg of zinc per day over time have been associated with lowering serum copper levels. Higher doses of 150 to 450 mg per day have resulted in altered iron function, reduced immune function, and lower levels of HDL cholesterol (the good cholesterol).

SUPPLEMENT CONSIDERATIONS: There are very few concerns with taking zinc as a supplement *if* you stay within the upper limit. I generally recommend taking a multivitamin-mineral product that provides 100 percent of the DV. Zinc comes in many forms but the body uses it more easily in the (bis)glycinate, gluconate, and yeast-bound forms.

Zinc lozenges are inexpensive and good to have on hand during cold and flu season. Research shows that both zinc acetate and zinc gluconate are effective for reducing the severity and length of a cold. The only downside to taking the lozenges is that those containing 20 mg or more of zinc will often leave an unpleasant taste in your mouth and upset your stomach. Look for those that contain 5 to 10 mg per lozenge and take one every two to three hours for three days. Short-term use of higher levels of zinc is not a problem.

However, using a zinc nasal spray might be. There were a number of reports that people who used them lost their sense of smell, some permanently. I'd say skip it.

And remember, water is the best liquid for taking supplements. Taking your zinc with black coffee can reduce absorption by up to 50 percent!

PARTNER NUTRIENTS: When high supplemental doses of zinc are taken on an empty stomach, it inhibits the absorption of iron. The moral of this story is to take your iron and zinc with food! High doses of zinc over a prolonged period of time can lower copper levels in your body. That is why many multivitamins that provide 40 mg or more of zinc also contain small amounts of copper.

Zinc and vitamin A are partners when it comes to eye health. Without adequate zinc, symptoms of vitamin A deficiency can appear even if you are taking vitamin A supplements. One study showed significant increases in retinol (preformed vitamin A) in the body when doses of up to 30 mg per day of zinc were given for six months.

Large doses of calcium and magnesium may impair the absorption of trace minerals, such as zinc. They are best taken at least two hours apart. Riboflavin improves zinc absorption. These are perfect examples of why I think taking a basic multivitamin-mineral product that provides all of your vitamins and trace minerals is a great supplement seatbelt strategy!

SPECIAL POPULATIONS: Vegetarians, vegans, and pregnant or breastfeeding women should take a multiple vitamin-mineral supplement that provides at least the DV for zinc.

And there you have it, the minerals you need to maintain good health. After reading these last two chapters, I hope you have gained an appreciation, as well as insight into the powerful inter-relationship that exists between vitamins and minerals and how a deficiency in one can wreak havoc with others. It is why I believe that for most of us trying to improve and/or maintain our health, taking a multivitamin-mineral supplement makes good sense, even if you need to take a higher amount of a specific nutrient, such as vitamins B12 or D.

Go back and review Chapter 2 for some key items to look for on the supplement label and then compare the amount and form of vitamins and minerals on the label with what I've recommended in the chapters on vitamins and minerals. You should be well positioned now to find one that is right for you!

It's also really important that if you take prescription or over-the-counter medications, you carefully review Appendix 4, "Drug-Nutrient Depletions and Interactions." Many drugs can cause nutrient deficiencies, increasing your need for certain vitamin and minerals. And sometimes, it's important to avoid certain supplements or take your supplements at a different time than your medication.

If you have a health concern, make sure you review Appendix 5, "Supplements to Address Common Ailments." This will help you identify some of the nutrients that are not only most important for conditions, such as diabetes, asthma, or migraines, but also for your particular stage in life: adolescence, pregnancy, or elder years.

But we're not finished yet. I still have a few more supplements that are really important for you to know. They are not vitamins or minerals, some are essential and some are not, but all of them can play a role in improving and maintaining your health. Let's take a peek at a few of my top nutraceutical choices.

Chapter 5

Nutraceuticals

We've all heard of vitamins and minerals—and now you know just how crucial they are for health—and many of us are familiar with herbal remedies, such as chamomile or echinacea, but there are hundreds of supplements in the marketplace that don't fall into these categories. Because they are so diverse, they are often just lumped together into one category called nutraceuticals. Please note that there is no legal or regulatory definition for what constitutes a nutraceutical. It's just a term that allows us to talk about the universe of supplements that are not vitamins, minerals, or herbals.

The supplement aisles are overflowing with these products. Health magazines, talk shows, and websites are filled with sound bites about the newest and greatest this or that. There are some with evidence of safety and effectiveness, while many others are unfortunately more hype than hope. I understand why so many of my patients end up with dozens of supplement bottles, often not understanding what they are taking or why.

It's easy to become overwhelmed. In Chapter 7, I share some advice for sorting through all the conflicting and confusing information that's out there. When you hear health claims or read advertisements that sound too good to be true, go check a variety of reliable sources to see what they say (see Resources). This category is enormous and it would take an entire book just to scratch the surface. I'm not going to go through a long and lengthy list.

Instead, I'm going to focus on those products that I think you really should know about. Some, such as omega-3 fatty acids and choline, are essential to your health, just like vitamins and minerals. Others—such as melatonin, alpha-lipoic acid, CoQ10, glucosamine, and SAMe—are made in the body but can also be taken in supplement form. These are the supplements that I often recommend to my patients and I want to share them with you.

ALPHA-LIPOIC ACID

Alpha-lipoic acid (also called thioctic acid) is a naturally occurring antioxidant that can be made in the body, though synthesis decreases as we age. It is also found in such foods as red meat, organ meats, spinach, broccoli, yams, carrots, beets, and yeast, though studies show that food sources don't really increase the levels found in our body. However, when taken as a supplement, alpha-lipoic acid can increase levels in both our blood and inside our cells.

Note: Alpha-lipoic acid is often written as "ALA," but I have used "LA" in this chapter so as to avoid confusion of this nutrient with alpha-linolenic acid, an omega-3 fatty acid also abbreviated as "ALA."

WHAT IT DOES: Nutritional research shows that LA may offer considerable benefit to our brain and nervous system for conditions ranging from sciatica to dementia. Since LA readily crosses the blood/brain barrier, its antioxidant effects may be particularly important in protecting the central nervous system from illness, disease, and DNA damage. Thus, it may play a role in helping protect us against Alzheimer's dementia and Parkinson's disease. One small double-blinded, placebo controlled 12-month study published in 2014 in the *Journal of Alzheimer's Disease* found that the combination of fish oil (975 mg of EPA and 675 mg of DHA) and LA (600 mg) slowed both cognitive and functional decline in people with dementia. There is also some evidence that when taken in combination with medications used to treat dementia, it further slows progression. Clearly, we are only in the very early stages of research, and neurodegenerative diseases are complex, but based upon what we know so far, LA may play an important role in the healthy aging of our brain.

Studies also show that LA may have a beneficial effect on blood sugar and alleviate some of the complications of diabetes. In a 2014 review published in the journal *Expert Opinion on Pharmacotherapy,* the authors summarized the data showing that randomized, double-blinded, placebo-controlled clinical trials have found LA to be both safe and effective for the treatment of diabetic neuropathy, helping to improve the numbness, tingling, and loss of muscle strength that accompanies the disorder. While the drug pregabalin (Lyrica) acts more quickly than LA to relieve pain, studies show that they are otherwise therapeutically equivalent. And given that people with diabetes are at increased risk for both Alzheimer's and vascular dementia, I personally believe that LA is a very important supplement for diabetics.

LA has been found to chelate toxic heavy metals, such as lead and mercury, enhancing their elimination from the body. In a world that is becoming increasingly toxic, that might make LA an important protective agent. There is also evidence that LA protects the liver, reducing the fibrosis that can develop due to injury.

WHO MIGHT BENEFIT FROM SUPPLEMENTING: Diabetics, particularly those that might be showing any signs of neuropathy (tingling, numbness, burning sensations), as well as people with a family history of dementia or other neurodegenerative diseases and anyone aged 65 or older may want to consider supplementing with LA.

HOW MUCH SHOULD YOU TAKE: 200 to 400 mg/day for most uses, 600 mg two times per day in cases of neuropathy or cognitive decline.

SAFETY: Oral doses of up to 2,400 mg per day in adults have not shown any serious adverse effects, but doses of 1,200 mg per day or higher can cause your urine to have a strange smell. A small

℞ RX FROM DR. LOW DOG
Alpha-Lipoic Acid and Healthy Aging

I've had the pleasure of meeting and listening to Dr. Bruce Ames, an emeritus professor of biochemistry and molecular biology at the University of California, Berkeley, who has done extensive research on mitochondria and aging. He found that if you want to maintain a healthy heart, brain, and nervous system, there is probably no better combination than LA and acetyl-l-carnitine (ALCAR), another potent antioxidant. These partner to enhance the energy production of the mitochondria, the powerhouse of our cells (see more about mitochondria under "CoQ10," page XXX). After listening to his lectures, I think many elders would benefit from taking a supplement that provides 500 to 1500 mg of ALCAR in addition to alpha-lipoic acid.

number of people have reported allergic reactions (hives, itching) when taking LA. When taking higher doses (1,200 mg or more per day), make sure that you are also taking a multivitamin that contains biotin, as LA can interfere with its absorption.

SUPPLEMENT CONSIDERATIONS: LA must be taken 30 minutes before meals for optimal absorption. If this upsets your stomach, which it has done in some of my patients, take it with a small amount of food. Supplements generally contain a mix of both forms of LA: R-alpha-lipoic acid and S-alpha-lipoic acid. While R-alpha-lipoic acid is better absorbed and more active, the research has almost all been conducted on the combination.

DRUG INTERACTIONS: If you have diabetes, be aware that LA might lower your blood sugar levels, so you might have to adjust your medications. LA *may* (theoretically) reduce the effectiveness of thyroid medications. As with any antioxidant supplement, discuss the use of LA with your oncologist before using while undergoing chemotherapy or radiation treatment.

CHOLINE

While choline is not technically a vitamin, in 1998, the Institute of Medicine (IOM) recognized it as an essential nutrient necessary for the structural integrity of cell membranes, proper liver function, heart health, synthesis of the neurotransmitter acetylcholine, the prevention of birth defects during pregnancy, and the healthy development of the brain and nervous system of young children. Given its importance to our health, it's disturbing that according to data from the 2007–2008 NHANES study, roughly 90 percent of Americans fail to meet the adequate intake for choline. Even worse, up to 40 percent of us may have a common gene variation that further increases our need for choline!

WHAT IT DOES: Choline is part of the brain's messaging system and is critical for the production of neurotransmitters, such as acetylcholine, that play a key role in memory, cognition, and muscle control. Clearly, choline is important across the lifespan, but I want to talk about its importance in pregnancy first. Like folic acid, choline plays a role in preventing birth defects, but it also appears to provide the child lifelong protection against anxiety and exaggerated responses to stressors. Given the state of today's world, even a small degree of protection may prove invaluable. Unfortunately, many pregnant women fall short of what they need. One study of 274 pregnant women in Boston published in 2014 in the *Public Health Nutrition* journal found that 95 percent had suboptimal intake of choline. Breastfed babies have a high need for choline in their mothers' milk to ensure brain development in areas involved with thought and memory. The FDA requires that choline be included in infant formula. Most prenatal supplements *do not contain choline.* So where is the choline going to come from in a breastfeeding mother? I cannot stress how important choline is in pregnancy, while breastfeeding and during early childhood.

Another beneficiary of choline is the liver, a vitally important organ with many jobs, including detoxification. Nonalcoholic fatty liver disease (NAFLD) is a condition where fat is deposited in the liver for reasons other than excessive alcohol use. It is the most common liver disorder in Western countries, affecting up to 30 percent of Americans, including children. It is more common in people who are overweight or have diabetes, high-cholesterol, or high triglycerides. High-fructose diets are also strongly associated with NAFLD, as are diets that are deficient in . . . yes, you guessed it: choline. Choline is involved in transporting fat and cholesterol away from the liver to tissues that need them. A deficiency in choline can cause fat to build-up in the liver and may also increase the risk for liver cancer by making it harder for the liver to protect us from carcinogenic substances in our diet and in the environment. The adequate intake for choline set by the Institute of Medicine is actually based upon the level needed to prevent liver damage. I find it kind of scary that 90 percent of us aren't getting enough in our diet!

Like folate and vitamin B12, choline also works to prevent the buildup of homocysteine in the blood, which can lead to cardiovascular disease. There is increasing evidence that choline also helps modulate inflammation in the body, so it might help prevent a multitude of chronic conditions.

Based on the Framingham Heart Study and the Nurses' Health Study, roughly 25 percent of Americans have diets and blood levels *very low* in this nutrient. Many people have not only upped their intake of sugary carbs but have also cut back on eggs and organ meats, two major sources of choline. Two hard-boiled eggs provide between 250 and 300 mg of choline, while 3 ounces of panfried beef liver yields 400 mg. Other good sources include soy lecithin granules (3 tablespoons provide 450 mg), wheat germ (1 cup provides 202 mg), and firm tofu (1 cup provides about 70 mg). In contrast, broccoli and cauliflower provide 82 and 177 mg *per pound,* respectively. Honestly, how many Americans are chowing down on beef liver, lecithin, or cups of wheat germ? It's not hard to see why we are choline deficient!

WHO MIGHT BENEFIT FROM SUPPLEMENTING: Pregnant and breastfeeding women should increase their consumption of choline-rich foods and look for a prenatal multivitamin-mineral supplement that contains the DV of choline. Those who are obese, diabetic, have fatty liver disease, are over the age of 65, or who consume more than two servings of alcohol per day should consider supplementation. I strongly recommend you consider supplementing with choline if your diet does not include eggs or organ meats!

HOW MUCH SHOULD YOU TAKE: Look for a supplement that provides 400 to 500 mg per day of choline.

AI: Men: 550 mg   Women: 425 mg
                            Pregnancy: 450 mg
                            Breastfeeding: 550 mg

UL: 3.5 grams/day for adults

SUPPLEMENT CONSIDERATIONS: Choline is available in supplemental form as choline bitartrate, choline chloride, phosphatidylcholine (lecithin), and cytidine 5'-diphosphate choline (CDP-choline), a form of choline said to more easily cross the blood-brain barrier. Make sure you are taking choline with other B-vitamins, particularly pantothenic acid, which is needed to convert choline to acetylcholine.

DRUG INTERACTIONS: None identified.

WARNING!
Don't Exceed the UL of Choline

Exceeding the upper limit (3,500 mg per day) of choline can lead to low blood pressure, diarrhea, and fishy-smelling body odor that results from the buildup of trimethylamine, a metabolic by-product of choline.

COENZYME Q10

Coenzyme Q10 (CoQ10), also known as ubiquinone, is a fat-soluble antioxidant that can be both synthesized by the body and consumed in foods, primarily fish, organ meats (including liver, kidney, and heart), and the germ layer of whole grains.

WHAT IT DOES: Could CoQ10 be a modern-day fountain of youth? Some scientists believe that CoQ10, along with LA and acetyl-l-carnitine, may help us age better and perhaps even live longer. This hypothesis is based upon the mitochondrial theory of aging. Mitochondria are the energy-producing structures within our cells. Some researchers believe that aging occurs when these powerhouses are damaged. CoQ10 is necessary for the proper function of mitochondria and is highly concentrated in the heart, liver, and pancreas.

I'd like to start my discussion with a discussion of the beneficial effects CoQ10 has on the heart. Studies show that when CoQ10 is taken alongside medication for the treatment of heart failure, it improves an individual's quality of life and such symptoms as shortness of breath and leg swelling, while decreasing the number of hospitalizations. CoQ10 has been approved in Japan for the treatment of heart failure since 1974. Small studies have also shown that when people with angina, or chest pain, take CoQ10, it can increase their exercise tolerance. CoQ10 may be particularly helpful for those who have suffered a heart attack. Some studies suggest that early supplementation may reduce the risk of having or dying from another heart attack. A 2011 review in the journal *Atherosclerosis* found that CoQ10 significantly improves the health of function of our arteries, which may reduce the risk of atherosclerosis. And finally, a 2007 meta-analysis of 12 studies published in the *Journal of Human Hypertension* found that CoQ10 lowers systolic blood pressure by up to 17 mm/Hg and diastolic blood pressure by up to 10 mm/Hg—not bad!

Your body uses the same metabolic machinery to make CoQ10 as it does to make cholesterol, and so statin drugs, taken to lower cholesterol, also lower CoQ10. Statins often make people feel tired and muscles feel weak. It was thought that these side effects could be due to low levels of CoQ10, which is why many physicians recommend supplementation while on these medications. However, clinical trials have generally failed to show that taking 100 to 200 mg per day of CoQ10 works any better than placebo for relieving statin-induced muscle pain and weakness.

As I've mentioned before, the brain is highly susceptible to oxidative stress and this may increase the risk for neurological disorders. CoQ10 is often recommended for patients with Parkinson's disease and dementia. There is some evidence that high doses (1,200–2,400 mg per day) may slow the functional decline in people with early Parkinson's disease when taken for at least 16 months; however, the beneficial effects were small. As for dementia, a 2014 study, published in the journal *Atherosclerosis,* reported that coenzyme Q10 levels are inversely correlated with the development of dementia. Higher levels appear protective. This is consistent with basic science and animal studies, but there are currently no rigorous clinical trials to determine whether supplementing with CoQ10 will delay the onset or slow the progression of dementia in humans.

CoQ10 is FDA approved as an "orphan drug" (a drug that is subsidized to treat rare diseases) for Huntington's disease. Currently a five-year randomized controlled trial is under way to compare the effects of 2400 mg/d of CoQ10 to placebo in patients with this rare inherited and horrific neurodegenerative disorder.

CoQ10 is beneficial for the prevention of migraines at doses of 100 mg taken three times per day. In fact, it was given a "strong recommendation" for migraine prophylaxis from the Canadian Headache Society. Some research indicates that migraines occur, in part, due to mitochondrial dysfunction.

There is evidence that low levels of CoQ10 may increase the risk for periodontal disease. When taken orally or applied topically, it reduces gingival (gum) bleeding and plaque. I've had dental colleagues as well as patients tell me they have found it to be very effective in cases of periodontitis, when used in conjunction with good dental care. One study found that 100 mg per day increased salivation in patients with dry mouth. There are now several toothpastes and oral care products that contain CoQ10.

Lastly, there is some research suggesting that CoQ10 may help improve sperm quality in men with infertility.

WHO MIGHT BENEFIT FROM SUPPLEMENTING: Those who have heart failure, high blood pressure, or migraines, or who are taking statins, tricyclic antidepressants, or beta-blockers (all of which can lower CoQ10 levels) should consider supplementation. For neurological disorders, such as Parkinson's disease, talk to your neurologist about the pros and cons of taking high doses of CoQ10.

HOW MUCH SHOULD YOU TAKE: Generally 100 to 300 mg per day is adequate for most conditions, though much higher doses are used for Parkinson's disease and other neurological disorders.

SUPPLEMENT CONSIDERATIONS: One of the key limitations with CoQ10 has been poor bioavailability. It not only has to be absorbed but it has to get inside the cell to do its job. At this time, I recommend ubiquinol, which evidence shows is more bioavailable than other forms. For optimal absorption, take with a fatty meal and take in divided doses. That means it is better to take 150 mg with breakfast and with dinner than 300 mg at once.

DRUG INTERACTIONS: CoQ10 may reduce the effectiveness of blood-thinning medications, such as warfarin (Coumadin). Please talk to your health-care provider before supplementing.

SAFETY: Doses of up to 2400 mg per day have been well tolerated in clinical trials lasting more than one year. Some people note that higher doses (>600 mg per day) cause heartburn, digestive upset, and headaches.

GLUCOSAMINE AND CHONDROITIN

Glucosamine and chondroitin are two naturally occurring substances found within the cartilage that cushions our joints, where they help to maintain joint integrity and flexibility. The combination of these two substances is commonly used for the treatment of osteoarthritis (OA).

WHAT IT DOES: Glucosamine and chondroitin are involved in the production of compounds used to build tendons, ligaments, and the fluid that surrounds the joints. Both have been shown to reduce inflammation and promote the synthesis of collagen, a substance that provides structural support for connective tissue in joints.

In spite of their popularity, there is a constant debate about the effectiveness of glucosamine and chondroitin. However, the majority of high-quality clinical trials have shown a beneficial effect for the *combination* of glucosamine sulfate (GS) or glucosamine hydrochloride (GH) and chondroitin sulfate (CS) in relieving the pain and improving the function of arthritic joints. Studies that used glucosamine or chondroitin alone did not show the same benefit. The controversy over the potential benefit for this over-the-counter aid for arthritis has really been rather tragic in my opinion, given how many people suffer with this condition. The alternatives we have to offer our patients—ibuprofen, celecoxib (Celebrex), acetaminophen—are all associated with adverse effects when taken continuously over time. What's more, none of these drugs has actually been shown to slow the progression of OA, yet there is evidence that the combination of glucosamine and chondroitin does.

Let's look at some of the recent research. A six-month, multi-center, randomized, double-blinded, European trial, whose results were published in 2014 in the prestigious *Annals of Rheumatic Diseases,* found that the combination of 1,500 mg GH and 1,200 mg CS per day was comparable to 200 mg per day of celecoxib for reducing pain, stiffness, and functional limitation in patients with painful knee OA. This is consistent with the Glucosamine-Chondroitin Arthritis Intervention Trial (GAIT) that failed to find any benefit for GH or CS alone but did find significant benefit for the *combination* in those with moderate-to-severe knee pain. In both studies, celecoxib worked more quickly, outperforming the combination for the first four months, but at six months, both interventions were equally effective.

Not only does the combination of glucosamine and chondroitin relieve pain over time, it also appears to slow the progression of the disease, which is good news for anyone wanting to put off a knee replacement! In 2014, the National Institutes of Health Osteoarthritis Initiative found that those taking the combination of GS and CS had less loss of cartilage in their knees over the two-year period, as viewed on MRI, compared to those taking analgesic medications. This finding was corroborated by a double-blinded, randomized, placebo-controlled Australian study published in 2014 in the *Annals of Rheumatic Diseases* that included 605 patients with knee OA. GS plus CS resulted in a statistically significant reduction of joint space narrowing compared to placebo. This effect was *not* seen in the treatment groups taking only glucosamine or chondroitin.

I want to stress that glucosamine and chondroitin are slow-acting agents. Significant relief is typically not seen for the first four months. You may need to take your analgesic medications during this time, but don't stop taking the supplements. The evidence that shows this combination can slow the progression of OA makes it worth using, given its safety and relatively low cost.

WHO MIGHT BENEFIT FROM SUPPLEMENTING: Anyone with joint pain due to aging and/or osteoarthritis and/or trauma should consider taking the combination of GS and CS. The earlier the better!

HOW MUCH SHOULD YOU TAKE: Take 1,500 mg per day of glucosamine sulfate and 1,200 mg chondroitin sulfate in two or three divided doses. Remember, the studies show that the longer you take the supplements, the greater the benefit.

SUPPLEMENT CONSIDERATIONS: While both glucosamine sulfate and glucosamine hydrochloride have both been studied, experts generally consider the sulfate form to be more effective. Studies consistently show that the combination is superior to either supplement taken alone.

DRUG INTERACTIONS: Taking glucosamine and chondroitin with blood thinners, such as warfarin (Coumadin), *may* increase the risk of bleeding so make sure you talk to your health-care provider *before* taking the supplement.

SAFETY: Glucosamine sulfate is found in the shells of shellfish (such as shrimp, lobster and crab), which are commonly used as a source for dietary glucosamine supplements. Although it is unlikely that someone would be allergic to glucosamine, as it is the shell that is used, not the meat protein, those with severe allergic reactions to shellfish should still exercise caution. Chondroitin is manufactured principally from bovine cartilage. For those that are vegetarian, some GH products in the marketplace are derived from corn but I am not currently aware of any vegetarian chondroitin supplements.

MELATONIN

Melatonin is a hormone secreted by the brain's pineal gland as well as by cells in the GI tract. While much of the focus has been on the role melatonin plays in maintaining our sleep-wake cycle, it also acts as an antioxidant, anti-inflammatory, pain reliever, and antidepressant. In addition, melatonin protects the GI tract and nervous system and assists in the regulation of blood sugar. It may even help protect us against certain cancers.

WHAT IT DOES: One of the primary roles for melatonin is maintaining our 24-hour circadian rhythm. At sunset, your body's internal clock sounds the alarm, telling the pineal gland to secrete melatonin, signaling the body that it is dark. In response, your body temperature begins to fall and you start to feel sleepy. As dawn begins to break, melatonin is suppressed, your body temperature starts to rise and you awaken. This biological process has been happening since the beginning of time.

For millennia, humans have predominantly relied on candles and fire for their light at night. These light sources had very little impact on our circadian rhythm. That's because not all wavelengths of light have the same impact on melatonin. Blue light, such as that from the sun and many artificial lights, is the strongest inhibitor of melatonin. You want melatonin to be suppressed during the daytime, and in fact, spending time outdoors during the day often helps people sleep better at night. However, many of us work indoors under artificial lights that have far less intensity than natural sunlight, so our melatonin is not fully suppressed during the day. And we wonder why we feel sleepy! Then we go home, turn the television and lights on, exposing ourselves until bedtime to blue light that suppresses our melatonin, and then we wonder why can't fall asleep. We have effectively turned our day and night upside down.

Given all the beneficial effects for melatonin, its chronic suppression may have significant adverse effects on our health. There are many things you can do to restore your own natural production of melatonin. I recommend using a dawn simulator to waken in the morning. Roughly 60 to 90 minutes before the time you are supposed to wake up, the light begins to slowly increase its glow, mimicking sunrise. Studies have shown dawn simulation and bright light therapy in the morning can help improve/prevent both seasonal and nonseasonal depression. Position your desk near a window at work and/or make sure that you get outside in natural light for at least 30 minutes midday. Start dimming the lights at home roughly 90 minutes before bedtime. Turn off the television and computer at least 60 minutes before bedtime (these both emit blue light). If these measures don't help, you might want to consider melatonin.

Melatonin, when taken several *hours* before sleep, can shorten the time it takes to fall asleep, as well as help you stay asleep.

Levels of melatonin should rise as evening sets in, peak in the middle of the night, and fall as morning approaches. People of all ages may benefit from its use. Children with autism spectrum disorder and ADHD are often troubled by poor sleep and studies show that melatonin can decrease the time it takes them to fall asleep and increase their total sleep time. A 2010 review published in the *Annals of Pharmacotherapy* concluded that melatonin is a well-tolerated and effective treatment option for children with ADHD who have chronic difficulty falling asleep. The studies included children 6 to 14 years old and melatonin doses ranging from 3 to 6 mg that were administered within a few hours of a scheduled bedtime. Our natural production of melatonin may decline with age. In Europe, sustained-release melatonin is approved for adults aged 55 and older who have primary insomnia.

Melatonin enhances dreaming. In fact, vivid dreaming is the number one side effect reported for the supplement. I believe many Americans are not only sleep deprived but also dream deprived. Dreams are necessary for our mental health, helping us to consolidate our memories, process our emotions, and wrestle through conflicts in our lives. Many indigenous cultures place great value on dreams. The aboriginal peoples of Australia believe that dreamtime is actually more important than our waking lives. Thus, melatonin's side effect of intensified dreaming could be good for us.

Let's step back for a moment and look at how we make melatonin. It starts with tryptophan, an essential amino acid that humans must get in their diet. Primary sources include meat, poultry, dairy, oats, soybeans, and seeds. Tryptophan can go down one of two pathways: It can be metabolized to kynurenine and then nicotinamide, a form of niacin (remember from the story of pellagra, page XX?). The other pathway leads to the production of 5-HTP, serotonin, and then melatonin. This is important. If your diet is low in niacin, your body will divert tryptophan to make this essential vitamin—at the expense of making serotonin and melatonin. You must also have plenty of vitamin B6 on board, as it is required to convert tryptophan to serotonin. And newer research shows that the enzyme that converts tryptophan to serotonin is activated by vitamin D! But according to the CDC, more than 30 million Americans are deficient in B6 and 66 million have insufficient levels of vitamin D! Are you beginning to see why so many people are feeling tired and depressed and are not sleeping well? And why I recommend that everyone take a basic multivitamin-mineral supplement?

While we are all familiar with the role of serotonin in mood (think of all the antidepressants that increase serotonin levels in the brain), melatonin also appears to play a role. For many women with breast cancer, difficulty sleeping, depression, and anxiety are common. A 2014 Danish study published in the journal *Breast Cancer Research and Treatment* randomized 54 women diagnosed with breast cancer and without depression to receive 6 mg of melatonin or placebo starting one week before their cancer surgery for a total of three months. The results were dramatic, with only 11 percent of women in the melatonin group experiencing depression versus 45 percent in the placebo group. Interestingly, research published in 2014 in the journal *Menopause* found that the later melatonin peaks in women going through menopause (perimenopause), the greater their anxiety. And the length of melatonin secretion mattered greatly. Longer periods of melatonin secretion were significantly associated with better quality of life. This is consistent with an older double-blinded placebo-controlled study that found taking 3 mg of melatonin at night for six months significantly improved symptoms of depression in perimenopausal and postmenopausal women.

WARNING!
Take Depression Very Seriously

Please note that self-care is appropriate for mild forms of depression, but if you are suffering from more severe depression, *you should not rely on over-the-counter supplements.*

Melatonin not only improves sleep quality but it may also help certain pain conditions, such as fibromyalgia, pelvic pain, irritable bowel syndrome, and even migraines. A 2014 study published in the *BMC Pharmacology & Toxicology* evaluating women with fibromyalgia (a chronic condition with musculoskeletal pain and fatigue) found that melatonin alone or in combination with the drug amitriptyline was superior to amitriptyline alone for relieving pain. Over the years I have used melatonin as part of an integrative treatment strategy for patients with fibromyalgia and have found that with continued use, it can raise the pain threshold and improve sleep.

Endometriosis, a condition where cells that normally line the uterus migrate to other places, is associated with chronic recurring pelvic pain in women. It affects more than six million women in the U.S. and treatment options are limited. Many women rely heavily on over-the-counter or prescription pain relievers. A growing body of basic science has shown that melatonin may be effective for relieving the pain of endometriosis. A double-blinded placebo-controlled trial randomized 40 women with endometriosis to either placebo or 10 mg of melatonin for eight weeks. The results published in the journal *Pain* in 2013 were very impressive. Compared to placebo, melatonin reduced daily pain scores by 39.8 percent, menstrual pain by 38 percent, while improving sleep quality, and reducing the need for analgesics by 80 percent.

This dose of melatonin is higher than what is typically used. I've found that women with chronic pelvic pain often do well on a 30-day trial of 5 mg melatonin two hours before bedtime.

Conventional medicine has limited treatment options available for treating irritable bowel syndrome (IBS), which affects roughly 10 to 15 percent of Americans. A 2014 review in the *World Journal of Gastroenterology* found that all clinical studies consistently showed melatonin, usually at a dose of 3 mg taken in the evening, improved abdominal pain in people with IBS. Let's dive a little deeper into this melatonin-gut relationship.

Because the pineal gland gets most of the credit for melatonin production, many people are unaware that cells in the GI tract produce large quantities of both serotonin and melatonin. Melatonin plays a major role in protecting the lining of the stomach and small intestine, and is found in very high concentrations in the large intestine and rectum, where it helps regulate gut motility and reduce abdominal cramping. This helps explain, in part, why it can be beneficial for IBS. It has been reported that low levels of melatonin may increase the risk for type 2 diabetes. Recently, scientists have found that cells in the pancreas also make melatonin. The pancreas is responsible for secreting the hormones insulin and glucagon, which regulate blood sugar levels.

Another important area of research is the use of melatonin for the prevention and treatment of gastroesophageal reflux (GERD). As melatonin levels rise, two things happen: The production of stomach acid is dialed back and the sphincter between your stomach and esophagus is tightened, preventing any upward flow of stomach acid. A very well-done study published in 2010 in *BMC Gastroenterology* showed that in just four weeks, patients with GERD taking 3 mg of melatonin before bedtime got very significant relief, and at the eight-week mark, there was no difference between the effectiveness of melatonin and Prilosec: All participants had complete relief of their symptoms. Considering all the troublesome side effects of proton pump inhibitors (PPIs), and the fact that in these studies, melatonin tightened the esophageal sphincter while the PPIs did not, my advice is to do a six- to eight-week trial of melatonin before taking a PPI if you have mild-to-moderate symptoms of GERD, or heartburn.

People who have diabetes often have poor gut motility—in other words, food doesn't move through their digestive system speedily. This can cause reflux, poor absorption of nutrients and medications, and GI symptoms such as gas, bloating, nausea, constipation, and diarrhea. Anyone with poor gut motility due to diabetes and/or GI disorders or chronic stress may find that melatonin alleviates GI problems along with making it easier to fall asleep without being bothered by heartburn.

Finally, I would like to just give a nod to the growing body of data suggesting that melatonin may help reduce the risk of certain cancers. An extensive review published in May 2015 in the *Journal of Pineal Research* reported that melatonin appears to inhibit the growth, invasion, and spread of cancer cells. Specifically the authors made a case for the protective effect in gastrointestinal cancers. In 2014, researchers reported in the journal *Oncology Letters* that melatonin may be particularly protective against breast cancer. There is much more work to do before we know whether melatonin has a place in cancer prevention or cancer survival. Yet, the science is sound and early research promising. Many of my integrative oncology colleagues routinely recommend it, especially for their patients with breast cancer.

WHO MIGHT BENEFIT FROM SUPPLEMENTING: Anyone who has difficulty falling asleep, suffers from heartburn, has mild symptoms of depression with poor sleep, fibromyalgia, diabetes, or irritable bowel syndrome, may benefit from a trial of melatonin. Plus, many medications both prescription and over-the-counter, interfere with the production of melatonin. Check Appendix 4, "Drug-Nutrient Depletions and Interactions," to see whether this pertains to you.

HOW MUCH SHOULD YOU TAKE: Melatonin comes in doses as low as .03 mg and as high as 20 mg. Based upon my own clinical experience and the scientific research, the optimal dosage range for people aged six or older is 1 to 6 mg taken roughly 2 hours before bedtime. I generally recommend, and personally take, 3 mg.

SUPPLEMENT CONSIDERATIONS: There are two points I want to stress: when to take melatonin and what form to use. Most people take it like a sleeping pill, meaning they swallow the pill, crawl into bed, and then wonder why they are still awake an hour later! *You must take it approximately two hours before bedtime* to mimic the natural secretion pattern of melatonin. Sometimes, this won't be feasible—for instance, if you're out late running errands or have an evening activity planned. However, you should try to take it around the same time most evenings to maintain your internal clock. Both fast-acting and sustained-release preparations are available. Some people who have a hard time staying asleep prefer the sustained-release preparation, but the fast-acting works well for just about everyone else and is best if you are dealing with heartburn.

DRUG INTERACTIONS: Taking melatonin with other sleeping medications may intensify their effects.

SAFETY: Studies have failed to show any serious adverse effects with melatonin even when taken for up to one year. It doesn't suppress your own production of melatonin and there is no rebound insomnia when you discontinue its use. Talk to your health-care provider before using melatonin if you are pregnant, breastfeeding, or being treated for cancer—and before using in a child under the age of six.

OMEGA-3 FATTY ACIDS

Humans are able to make most of the fats we need. However, there are two essential fatty acids we must get in our diet: linoleic acid, an omega-6 fatty acid, and alpha-linolenic acid, an omega-3 fatty acid. Our body needs these essential fatty acids to make and maintain the membranes that surround all of our cells, regulate our immune and inflammatory responses, promote wound healing and healthy skin and hair, regulate metabolism, and support the structure and function of our brain, nervous system, eyes and bones, particularly during fetal and early childhood development.

Are you wondering what makes something an omega-6 or omega-3 fatty acid? It's just chemistry. An omega 6-fatty acid has its first double bond located between the sixth and seventh carbon atom from the methyl end of its fatty acid chain. An omega-3 fatty acid has its first double bond, you guessed it, located between the third and fourth carbon atom. We need both omega-6 and omega-3 fatty acids. Contrary to what you might have read, omega-6 fatty acids are not bad for you. You must have some in your diet. It's just that most Americans get far too much omega-6 in their diets because so many of our processed foods are made with vegetable oils derived from corn, safflower, sunflower, and soybeans. Omega-6 fats play an important role in stimulating inflammation, which is extremely important when you are injured or ill—you need it to mobilize your immune cells. However, too much omega-6 can cause excessive amounts of inflammation, which has been associated with heart disease, diabetes, arthritis, osteoporosis, and cancer.

Omega-3 fatty acids have many roles in the body but one important job is to turn off inflammation. Unfortunately, the American diet is woefully lacking in omega-3s, which is why I want to focus the rest of my discussion on them. There are three omega-3 fatty acids you should be familiar with: ALA (mentioned previously), eicosapentaenoic acid (EPA) and docosahexaenonic acid (DHA).

Let's start with alpha-linoleic acid (ALA), the most common omega-3 fatty acid in the American diet. It is found primarily in nuts (walnuts are the richest source), canola oil, and flax, chia, and hemp seeds, as well as in Brussels sprouts and green leafy vegetables, such as kale. ALA is the only true *essential* omega-3 fatty acid—the one you have to get from your diet.

EPA and DHA can technically be synthesized in the body from ALA, which is why they are not considered "essential." However, humans can't make EPA and DHA very well from ALA. Let me give you an example. If you give a healthy man 1,000 mg of ALA, he can convert it to roughly 80 mg of EPA and 0 to 40 mg of DHA—not good at all. Young women do a better job because they have more estrogen, a hormone that helps with the conversion process. If you give a young woman 1,000 mg ALA, she can convert it to roughly 210 mg of EPA and 90 mg of DHA. That's better, but still not very good. Because babies absolutely require DHA for the development of their brain, nervous system, and eyes, there was likely a strong biological pressure to ensure that women were able to optimize their ability to convert plant sources of ALA to DHA. Unfortunately, after menopause, women have less estrogen and consequently, convert their ALA no better than men do. There also appear to be genetic differences in our ability to elongate ALA to EPA and DHA.

Are EPA and DHA that important? Absolutely. They are critical to the health of our cardiovascular system, brain, and eyes. They decrease inflammation, reduce our risk for certain cancers, are critical during fetal development, and may even help protect us from depression. That's why experts recommend eating fish two or three times per week. Fish are rich in EPA and DHA, premade and ready for our body to use—no conversion necessary. You can also find EPA and/or DHA in omega-3-enriched eggs, wild game, grass-fed beef, and certain seaweeds. Wherever you get your omega-3s, one thing is for sure: You need them!

WHAT IT DOES: Omega-3 fatty acids, along with omega-6 fatty acids, are key structural components in our cell membranes, where they act to stabilize and protect them from damage. This is particularly important for the cells in our brain, eyes, and nervous system, especially during pregnancy and our babyhood.

During the last trimester of pregnancy, neurological development is very rapid and omega-3s, particularly DHA, are concentrated in the baby's brain and eyes. Studies show that babies born to women who consumed fish or fish oil during pregnancy score higher on tests that assess intelligence, attention, and visual acuity. DHA may also reduce the risk of premature birth. In 2013, in a randomized, double-blinded, government-funded study of 350 pregnant women in Kansas City, published in the *American Journal of Clinical Nutrition,* when compared to placebo, women taking 600 mg of DHA per day during the last half of pregnancy had significantly fewer babies born prematurely or with a very low birth weight. That's a very important finding, given the risk to the baby if born too early and too small. There is also some evidence that higher maternal intake of DHA may offer some protection against allergies and asthma in the baby. Children continue to need a steady supply of DHA for at least the first two years of life to ensure the proper development and function of their central nervous system. DHA is added to infant formula, but the *level in breast milk depends exclusively on the mother's diet.*

Omega-3s may offer some additional protection for the mother during pregnancy. In a double-blinded, placebo-controlled trial, 64 African-American women between 16 and 24 weeks pregnant, living in a low-income urban environment, took either 450 mg per day of DHA or an identical placebo. The paper, published in 2014 in the journal of *Obstetrics and Gynecology,* reported that after controlling for life events and depression, women taking the DHA reported less stress and had lower blood levels of stress hormones during their last trimester compared to women taking the placebo. This is highly significant not only for the mother but because high levels of stress hormones during pregnancy may be detrimental to the baby.

In 2007, a European committee composed of more than 50 nutritional experts from the Perinatal Lipid Nutrition Group and Early Nutrition Programming unanimously recommended that all pregnant and lactating women consume a *minimum* of 200 mg DHA per day. This recommendation was supported by seven international scientific organizations. Eating fatty fish twice a week should provide this level of DHA. However, the committee endorsed the use of supplements for women who don't regularly eat fish. After reviewing the available studies, the committee found no evidence of adverse effects or outcomes for mothers or babies when mothers took up to 1,000 mg per day of DHA. Yet, in spite of the vast evidence of benefit and safety, studies repeatedly show that women in the U.S., Canada, and many European countries are not getting anywhere near the recommended levels of DHA in their diets. *This is one case when supplements absolutely make sense!*

Let's switch gears now and talk about the relationship between omega-3s and inflammation. Medications, such as aspirin, ibuprofen, or prednisone, have long been used to suppress inflammation. It was thought that suppressing inflammation was a useful strategy while waiting for the inflammation to fizzle out on its own. We didn't know that there might be an "off" switch. Well, it turns out that EPA and DHA are responsible for resolving inflammation, for turning it off and cleaning up any of the cellular debris that remains. Resolvins and protectins are molecules generated from omega-3s that orchestrate the timely resolution of inflammation in our body. The E-series resolvins are derived from EPA and the D-series resolvins are from, you guessed it, DHA. These resolvins also seem to be critically important for maintaining our mucosal barriers (such as the mucosal lining of the respiratory tract), and when they are low, we can experience more severe allergies and asthma. Protectins are derived only from DHA and protect our nerve tissue, brain, and eyes; they also interact with our immune cells. This new understanding of omega-3s may help explain why fish oil has shown benefit in patients with rheumatoid arthritis, asthma, and other inflammatory-driven diseases.

Much of the chronic disease we are experiencing is fueled by persistent low-grade inflammation, driven by many factors of modern living such as obesity, insulin resistance, a high-fructose diet, lack of physical activity, chronic stress, and poor sleep, to name a few. The term *inflammaging* is being used to describe the many diseases of old age such as heart disease, diabetes, and cognitive decline that are now being seen in younger and younger people. Increasing our intake of omega-3 fatty acids, as part of a holistic strategy, may help reverse or slow this premature aging process.

Earlier you saw how important DHA is during our early life. It remains so across our lifespan, especially as we move into our elder years. Low blood levels of DHA are associated with cognitive decline in healthy elders. A 2010 double-blinded placebo-controlled study published in the journal *Alzheimer's*

Dementia randomized 485 people with age-related cognitive decline to receive 900 mg of DHA or identical placebo for 24 weeks. The researchers found that DHA improved learning and memory scores, particularly immediate and delayed verbal recall. Similar effects were seen in a small 12-month study published in *Psychopharmacology* in 2013 that found fish oil with high concentrations of DHA significantly improved immediate and delayed verbal recall (both are measures of memory). There were no adverse effects in either study. Studies suggest omega-3 is probably most useful as a preventive agent or for those with very early cognitive decline, as the studies using EPA and/or DHA in

RX FROM DR. LOW DOG

R℞ Omega-3s and Brain Injury

Protectins derived from DHA offer considerable protection to the brain and central nervous system. Emerging science is demonstrating how DHA can help the brain heal after injury, or perhaps even more critical, protect the brain if it should become injured. I have had four concussions in my life that have all included loss of consciousness. The worst was when I was thrown from my horse and lost my short-term memory for almost seven hours. I don't recall any of it but needless to say, it scared both my family and the doctors caring for me. I've taken care of competitive athletes and military veterans, and I've seen the possible long-term outcomes of traumatic brain injury. That's why the evidence suggesting DHA may help the brain repair itself after injuries, such as stroke or concussion, intrigues me. Given the safety of fish oil supplements, anyone who may be at increased risk for head trauma should consider taking 1,000 mg of DHA every day.

those with Alzheimer's dementia have unfortunately not shown any significant benefit.

There is evidence that omega-3s may play an important role in mood. A fascinating 2014 report in the journal *Military Medicine* found moderate to strong evidence that higher levels of EPA and DHA are associated with a lower risk of clinical depression. They also noted that meta-analyses of randomized placebo-controlled trials provide moderate to strong evidence that when the supplement contained more than 50 percent EPA, there was a significant improvement in symptoms of depression. They even noted that there is modest evidence of clinical benefit for ADHD. Given the dramatic stressors our military men and women are under, increasing omega-3s in their diet and providing high quality marine omega-3s seems like a no-brainer to me.

Most people are aware that omega-3 fatty acids are good for the heart. And as of April 2015, it appears that the American Heart Association (AHA) agrees. On its website *(www.heart.org)* it says "omega-3 fatty acids benefit the heart of healthy people and those at high risk of—or who have—cardiovascular disease. Research has shown that omega-3 fatty acids decrease risk of arrhythmias (abnormal heartbeats), which can lead to sudden cardiac death. Omega-3 fatty acids also decrease triglyceride levels, slow the growth rate of atherosclerotic plaque and lower blood pressure (slightly)." The AHA recommends eating fatty fish at least two times per week and acknowledges that some people may need to take fish oil supplements.

WHO MIGHT BENEFIT FROM SUPPLEMENTING: Anyone who doesn't regularly consume fatty fish twice a week should supplement with fish oil. I believe the data clearly show that the vast majority of Americans do not get enough omega-3s in their diet. I also believe that it is the steady intake of these fatty acids over our lifetime that offers the best protection against chronic disease. The benefits you'll gain if you start taking fish oil at age 70, while still good, would not be near as great as if you started upping your intake of omega-3s in your 30s.

HOW MUCH YOU SHOULD TAKE: For most people, taking 400 to 800 mg of EPA and 200 to 500 mg of DHA per day, or three or four times per week is probably sufficient. Some

RX FROM DR. LOW DOG
Choosing the Right Fish

Most experts recommend eating 4 ounces of fatty fish twice a week. When choosing fish, make sure you learn which ones are high in omega-3s and low in mercury, dioxins, PCBs, or other contaminants. If you eat local fish, check with your state fish and wildlife department to determine if there are any advisories about which fish, lakes, and rivers may be contaminated. You can find that information online. In general, larger predatory fish are more likely to have higher levels of mercury and other toxins. The notable exception is salmon, which have a short life cycle. When it comes to avoiding mercury in seafood, my favorite source for information on which fish to favor is the seafood calculator on the Environmental Working Group website (*www. EWG.org*). You simply type in your age, gender, and weight—and indicate whether you have a heart condition—and it tells you which fish are highest in omega-3s, lowest in mercury, and safest for you to consume (and how often you can eat them). It also lets you know which fish sources are the most sustainable. Despite what you might have read, there are times when farm-raised fish are your best bet and times when wild is the only option that makes sense.

conditions, such as rheumatoid arthritis, or to lower elevated triglycerides requires doses of 2 to 3 grams of EPA and 1 to 2 grams of DHA.

SUPPLEMENT CONSIDERATIONS: In the U.S., fish oil manufacturers are doing a good job of removing mercury, PCBs, and other contaminants. But to be certain that you are getting a high-quality product, check to see whether it is approved by the International Fish Oil Standards Program, an organization that independently tests products for purity and quality *(www.nutra-source.ca/ifos)*. Click on the Consumer Reports tab and enter the brand and product you want to look up.

There's been a great deal of marketing around the different types of marine omega-3s. However, a 2014 study published in the journal *Lipids in Health and Disease* compared four different types: concentrated triglycerides, ethyl ester, whole salmon, and krill. Hands down, the concentrated triglycerides resulted in the most significant rise in blood EPA and DHA. That's the form I recommend.

Some fish oil capsules can be very large and difficult to swallow. Today's liquid fish oils bear no resemblance to the cod-liver oil I had as a child. I've done many taste tests with my physician students over the years in which I mixed some natural orange-flavored liquid fish oil into plain or vanilla yogurt. No fishy aftertaste, no burping, no pills to swallow, and I swear it tastes just like a Dreamsicle! I've yet to have a single person tell me that it wasn't a delightful way to take fish oil, especially when trying to give it to a picky 5-year old! There are companies that make delicious little gummies or pudding-like forms that can be taken on a spoon. My point is simply that you don't have to take pills if you don't want to. Always store your fish oil supplements in the refrigerator to keep them fresh.

Nonfish Omega-3s

For those who are vegetarian, vegan, or allergic to fish, there are several strategies you can use to up your omega-3 intake. You can add freshly ground flaxseeds to your diet, as they are rich in ALA, dietary lignans, and fiber. In fact, flax is one of the richest sources of dietary lignans, which offer significant protection against cancer. Purchase the seeds whole and grind as you use them. While you might enjoy their crunchy, nutty flavor, you have to grind them before use; otherwise, they pass through you essentially undigested and you won't get the benefit of its omega-3 fatty acids! Brown or golden seeds have the same nutritional benefits and contain roughly 800 mg of ALA per tablespoon of ground seeds. Aim for 2 tablespoons per day. Chia seeds also contain ALA but less than flax. They also don't have those powerhouse lignans. However, they don't need to be ground, are a great source of soluble fiber, and are easy to throw into smoothies and tea. You can also get omega-3s by adding walnuts and other nuts to salads. Beans, soy, cauliflower, broccoli, purslane, and other green leafy vegetables contain small amounts of ALA. If you consume eggs, pay the extra one or two dollars per dozen and buy free-range omega-3-enriched eggs. And if you drink milk, go for the omega-3-enriched variety.

As it can be hard to get enough DHA in your diet, especially during pregnancy and while breastfeeding, in these cases, you might want to consider taking a supplement containing DHA derived from microalgae. Other vegetarian sources of EPA and DHA are being investigated and will likely be on the market soon.

DRUG INTERACTIONS: While it is theoretically possible to have an increased risk of bleeding from taking fish oil with medications designed to prevent blood clots, this is likely only to happen with very high doses. (See "Safety," below.)

SAFETY: You may have heard that taking fish oil supplements can increase your risk for bleeding, but that hasn't really been born out. The European Food Safety Authority (EFSA) published its *Scientific Opinion Related to the Tolerable Upper Intake Level of EPA, DHA and DPA* in the *EFSA Journal* in 2012. The committee concluded that based upon more than 48 studies, "supplemental intakes of EPA and DHA combined of up to about 5g/day for up to two years, and up to about 7g/day for up to six months, do not increase the risk of spontaneous bleeding episodes or bleeding complications, even in subjects at high risk of bleeding (e.g., taking aspirin or anticoagulants)."

Men also ask me whether fish oil supplements increase their risk for prostate cancer. I am happy to report that in 2014, after a thorough review of the scientific evidence, the European Food Safety Authority concluded, "there is no evidence for a role of EPA and/or DHA intake in the development of prostate cancer."

PROBIOTICS

In and on our body are more than 100 trillion microorganisms. They inhabit our skin, nose, mouth, throat, gut, lungs, and genitourinary tract and play a vital role in maintaining our health. We have a symbiotic relationship with these microbes: We provide them a home and in return, they help us out by extracting and synthesizing vitamins and other nutrients from our food; regulating digestion, metabolism, and elimination; fine-tuning the immune system; preventing the overgrowth of harmful bacteria; and maintaining the integrity and barrier function of the intestinal wall. This complex community of microbes is collectively referred to as the microbiome.

Many things can disrupt our microbiome. Antibiotics, diets high in fructose, chronic stress, being born prematurely or by C-section, exposure to environmental toxins, consumption of meat from animals fed antibiotics, frequent use of nonsteroidal anti-inflammatories (such as ibuprofen or aspirin), prolonged use of PPIs, and even normal aging can perturb the delicate balance of these microbes. Hmm. I've just described most of America!

Probiotics are one way to restore and maintain a healthy microbiome. Probiotics are live bacteria and yeast, or "friendly" microbes that are found in certain foods or in supplements, which are particularly beneficial for our digestive tract. Here they decrease the number of "bad" bacteria that can cause infection or drive inflammation and increase the number of "good" bacteria that do all the jobs I mentioned above.

Although researchers have given us a whole new perspective on the beneficial effects of probiotics, people have been enjoying them in their food for millennia. You can find them in abundance in the traditional diets of Mediterranean, Middle Eastern, and Asian countries in the form of fermented milk, buttermilk, kefir, yogurt, some soft cheeses, pickled vegetables, miso, tempeh, and kimchi. I strongly encourage you to include these foods in your diet and you might also want to consider taking probiotics in supplement form, as well.

WHAT IT DOES: Our GI tract is an amazingly complex system. It has its own nervous system made up of more than 100 million neurons embedded within the gut wall stretching from the esophagus to the anus. This enteric nervous system produces neurotransmitters, hormones, and other compounds that are very similar to those found in the brain—in fact, roughly half of all our dopamine, 90 percent of the body's serotonin, and a considerable amount of melatonin are found in the gut. Because the digestive tract is constantly exposed to potentially harmful substances in our diet, between 70 and 80 percent of our immune cells are found here, producing more antibodies than all the rest of the body put together. The microbiome is actually a metabolically active organ that plays a key role in mediating the diverse and complex communication that exists between these three vitally important systems in our body: the gastrointestinal, immune, and nervous systems. Clearly, given its importance, we should all want to ensure that our internal ecology is in optimal shape.

How do we get all these bacteria in the first place? Well, let's go back to the beginning. When we are in our mother's womb, our GI tract is sterile. When we are born, we ingest and take in our mother's bacteria as we travel through the birth canal. It is *her* microflora that lays the foundation for *our* microbiome. Breastfeeding further stimulates and adds to our inner microbial population, as breast milk is rich in *Bifidobacteria*. *Bifidobacteria* plays an important role in helping our immune system learn to distinguish between dangerous and innocuous substances, reducing the risk for allergies. Children born by C-section do not have this initial exposure to the mother's rich store of healthy microorganisms in the birth canal. Even if the child is breastfed, babies born by C-section are at increased risk for milk and respiratory allergies, celiac disease, diabetes, and possibly obesity. It is thought that it is the alteration of their early microbial communities that either cause or contribute to the development of these problems.

Since we know that probiotics during early life are important for teaching the immune system that it should respond to dangerous bacteria but not to peanuts, it makes sense that early use of probiotics might help reduce the risk of allergies. And that is exactly what the evidence is showing: certain strains of probiotics can help reduce the risk of both allergies and eczema (atopic dermatitis). A meta-analysis, based on randomized controlled studies and published in the prestigious journal *Pediatrics* in 2013, concluded that children born to women who took probiotics during the latter part of pregnancy, and/or were given probiotics for the first six months of their lives, were significantly less likely to develop eczema and common childhood allergies. This is good news considering that these conditions affect 10 to 20 percent of all children! Probiotics may be even more important if a child was born by C-section.

Let's talk about antibiotics for a moment. While they can be lifesaving when used appropriately, they are overprescribed and can have serious long-term consequences to our health. Based upon his 30-plus years of research, Martin Blaser, M.D., director of the Human Microbiome Program at New York University (NYU), contends that the use of antibiotics in very young children poses one of the greatest risks to our long-term health because of their effect on the gut microbiome. He posits that it could be driving the increase in type 1 diabetes, the 50 percent increase in asthma among Americans from 2001 to 2009, the staggering numbers of people with food allergies, and the obesity epidemic. As someone familiar with ranching and farming, I know that low-dose antibiotics have long been used to increase the weight and growth of livestock. Is it such a stretch to think that early antibiotic exposure could increase the risk of obesity and metabolic syndrome in humans? I believe many factors are at play, but biologically, it makes sense. Most Americans have taken an average of 17 courses of antibiotics before they've celebrated their 21st birthday. This was one of the primary reasons I wrote *Healthy at Home*: so people could learn how to care for many common ailments without antibiotics.

Antibiotics don't just kill the "bad bugs." The rapid destruction of friendly organisms often leads to one of the most common side effects of taking antibiotics: diarrhea. Fortunately, taking probiotics can make a bad situation better. If you have to take antibiotics, make sure you start taking probiotics within 72 hours and continue to take them for at least three to six months. A 2012 meta-analysis published in the *Journal of the American Medical Association* reviewed 63 trials including almost 12,000 participants and found that taking probiotics resulted in a 42 percent reduction in the risk of developing antibiotic-associated diarrhea. Probiotics are useful for other causes of diarrhea, too. They have been shown to prevent diarrhea in children in daycare settings, reduce the severity and duration of infectious diarrhea, and prevent traveler's diarrhea. I recommend children in daycare and kindergarten take probiotics on a regular basis. Diarrhea can spread like wildfire in these settings!

When our gut ecology is out of balance, it can often result in constipation, gas, bloating, or "dumping syndrome" (loose bowels or diarrhea shortly after eating). These symptoms are often lumped together under the diagnosis of irritable bowel syndrome (IBS). Randomized studies have shown that probiotics, particularly *Bifidobacteria,* can help correct these symptoms by repopulating your intestinal tract with beneficial organisms. While the exact mechanism isn't understood, well-done clinical studies have found that probiotics can help quell the inflammation seen in Crohn's disease and ulcerative colitis. Because prolonged intestinal inflammation has been associated with an increased risk for colorectal cancer, researchers are currently investigating whether probiotics may play a protective role.

And quelling inflammation is important. We know that chronic inflammation contributes to cardiovascular disease, neurodegenerative disease, obesity, and even depression. A growing number of studies show that probiotics reduce inflammation throughout our body, not just in our GI tract. How is that possible? Well, as I said in the opening paragraphs, many things in our modern lives can disrupt the delicate and complex balance of our microbiome. This disruption leads to an increase in "bad bacteria," which increases inflammation and permeability in the intestine, a condition often referred to as "leaky gut." Our intestinal tract was designed to tightly regulate what stays in our intestine and what is released into our bloodstream. That's why there are tight junctions, or barriers, between the cells in our intestine. Our friendly bacteria act as guards at these tight junctions, signaling which substances are safe to go through and which ones should be denied entry. Unfortunately, when the bad bacteria outnumber the good, there are not enough soldiers to guard the gates. When fragments of bacterial cell walls or certain proteins from foods slip through and out into the bloodstream, they trigger a low-level inflammatory response throughout the body. Most of us probably have leaky gut to one degree or another, which is why I feel so strongly that essentially everyone would benefit from probiotics.

Finally, research also shows that probiotics can help prevent vaginal infections, give our respiratory system a boost against colds, and possibly even protect us against heavy metal toxicity. *Bottom line: Neglect your inner ecology at your own peril!*

WHO MIGHT BENEFIT FROM SUPPLEMENTING: I believe, essentially, that everybody needs to enrich their internal microbiome by upping their consumption of live-culture yogurt, kefir, and fermented foods. Beyond that, I think the following should consider supplementing: anyone with digestive problems; anyone who has taken or is taking antibiotics; people who have allergies, acute or chronic diarrhea, diabetes, cardiovascular disease, recurrent bladder infections, inflammatory disorders, or periodontal disease; children in daycare centers; people traveling where infectious diarrhea may be common, women during the last six weeks of pregnancy; and infants. *Hmm. Is there anyone I left out?*

HOW MUCH YOU SHOULD TAKE: When you buy them in supplement form, a probiotic capsule or tablet will contain millions or billions of microorganisms. How much you need varies based upon the species of probiotic. The following recommendations are based upon clinical studies and provide a range. See "Supplement considerations," page XXX, for guidelines on selecting the right types of probiotics or probiotic combinations for you.

For children up to 12 years of age:
Saccharomyces boulardii: 250 mg two times a day
Lactobacillus rhamnosus GG: 1 billion colony forming units 2 times a day

For people 12 years of age and older:
Saccharomyces boulardii; 500 mg twice a day
Lactobacillus acidophilus: 10 billion organisms 1–2 times per day
Lactobacillus rhamnosus GG: 10 billion organisms 1–2 times per day
Lactobacillus reuteri: 100 million organisms 1–2 times per day
Lactobacillus casei: 1–10 billion organisms once a day
Bifidobacterium infantis: 100 million organisms 1–2 times per day
Bifidobacterium bifidum: 1–3 billion organisms 1–2 times per day
Bifidobacterium lactis: 3–5 billion organisms 1–2 times per day

SUPPLEMENT CONSIDERATIONS: Probiotics contain live microorganisms. To preserve their effectiveness, most probiotics need to be refrigerated. I recommend supplements that also contain some prebiotics, substances that help promote the growth of healthy microorganisms already inhabiting your GI tract. These will usually appear on the label as fructo-oligosaccharides (FOS) or inulin. Which probiotic to choose depends on what health condition you are trying to address. Look for a product that provides at least one of the following species for:

Acute diarrhea: *L. GG, L. acidophilus, S. boulardii, B. lactis*

Preventing diarrhea: *L. reuteri, L. casei, L. GG, S. boulardii*

Antibiotic-associated diarrhea: *S. boulardii* and *L. GG*

Traveler's diarrhea: *S. boulardii* or *L. GG*

Irritable bowel syndrome: *B. infantis, B. animalis, B. lactis*

Inflammatory bowel disease: VSL #3, a combination probiotic product

Intestinal health: *B. lactis, B. infantis, L. plantarum, L. rhamnosus*

Obesity: *L. gasseri, L. rhamnosus, B. lactis*

Vaginal/urinary health: *L. rhamnosus, L. reuteri, L. plantarum, L. crispatus*

High cholesterol/blood sugar: *L. acidophilus, L. rhamnosus, L. paracasei, B. lactis, B. longum*

Health maintenance: combination of *Lactobacillus* and *Bifidobacterium* species along with prebiotics

Key to probiotic names:

B. animalis is *Bifidobacterium animalis*

B. infantis is *Bifidobacterium infantis*

B. lactis is *Bifidobacterium lactis*

B. longum is *Bifidobacterium longum*

L. acidophilus is *Lactobacillus acidophilus*

L. casei is *Lactobacillus casei*

L. crispatus is *Lactobacillus crispatus* (taken as vaginal suppository)

L. gasseri is *Lactobacillus gasseri*

L. GG is *Lactobacillus rhamnosus GG*
L. paracasei is *Lactobacillus paracasei*
L. plantarum is *Lactobacillus plantarum*
L. rhamnosus is *Lactobacillus rhamnosus*
L. reuteri is *Lactobacillus reuteri*
S. boulardii is *Saccharomyces boulardii*

DRUG INTERACTIONS: None known.

SAFETY: Probiotics are widely used and have been widely studied. They are considered quite safe for the general population. There is a small risk that people who are immune compromised due to disease or medication may be at risk for infection by taking probiotics. Talk to your health-care provider if you have any concerns about whether probiotics are right for you.

SAMe

SAMe (pronounced Sam-ee), short for S-adenosyl-l-methionine, is a naturally occurring compound in the body made from the amino acid methionine. SAMe is present in every cell of our body and is required for a whole host of activities, particularly when it comes to brain, liver, and joint health. SAMe was first identified in 1952 and since then has been studied for the treatment of depression, osteoarthritis, and liver disease. SAMe has been available as a prescription drug in some European countries for more than 35 years. It is sold as a dietary supplement in the U.S. and it is one nutraceutical that I believe has potential to improve the quality of life for many.

WHAT IT DOES: I learned about SAMe from one of my patients, Dora, almost 20 years ago. In her late 70s, Dora was living with rheumatoid arthritis and had a very sour disposition. She was on multiple medications and was wheelchair-bound. One day, her daughter brought her into the office for her appointment, and Dora could hardly control herself. "Show her the bottle. Show the doctor the bottle! Works better than anything they've ever given me." When her daughter showed me a bottle of SAMe, I admitted that I didn't really know anything about it. At which point Dora said, "Well, what do they teach you doctors?" Dora's hairdresser had told her about SAMe and suggested she try it. Within just a few weeks, she had less pain and felt less depressed. I was skeptical of the latter given our interaction that day! But over the next few months, I clearly watched the supplement dramatically improve her quality of life.

I've learned a lot about SAMe since then. And it is one of my go-to treatments for people living with depression and chronic pain. I've seen it work wonders. This shouldn't surprise us if we think about what it does in the body. SAMe is necessary for the production of the neurotransmitters: dopamine, serotonin, norepinephrine, and melatonin, which help us maintain a healthy mood, experience pleasure, and regulate our sleep-wake cycle. SAMe has been studied for the treatment of depression for decades, a condition for which it has been used in Europe for more than 30 years. SAMe readily crosses the blood-brain barrier, ensuring that it can increase brain levels of neurotransmitters. Studies have found that SAMe supplements are superior to placebo and equally as effective as prescription antidepressant medications in the treatment of depression.

I can't tell you the number of patients I've had over the years who've had great pain relief from supplementing with SAMe. I had one elder patient with fallen arches in her feet that had led to significant pain and arthritis. It was hard for her to walk even with special orthotic shoes. I started her on SAMe, telling her I wanted her to work her way slowly up to 600 to 800 mg per day. When she came back for her follow-up appointment with her husband six weeks later, they were both ecstatic about how well it was working. Her husband said, "I just didn't realize how much her feet were hurting her. She just seems so much happier now." I've heard similar reports from many patients over the years: SAMe relieves pain and eases depression.

A 2011 review published in the prestigious journal *Rheumatology* found consistent evidence for the effectiveness of SAMe in the treatment of osteoarthritis, an all-too-common pain condition in the U.S. Research shows that when used over the course of eight weeks, SAMe supplements provide the same pain relief as such drugs as celecoxib (Celebrex) and indomethacin. While SAMe reduces pain and improves function quickly, it is still important to take glucosamine or chondroitin to maintain the integrity of the joints over the long haul. I have also found that some of my patients with fibromyalgia have less pain, fatigue, and depression when taking SAMe.

Abdominal pain is common in children. When it is ongoing and tests and investigations are unable to find a source for the pain, it is called functional abdominal pain. Functional abdominal pain is one of the most common reasons children and teens are seen by GI doctors. Tricyclic antidepressants are generally used to treat the condition, but these medications have many side effects, including an increased risk for contemplating suicide. Pediatricians at the University of California, San Diego postulated that SAMe might be effective for this condition due to its dual effects as an antidepressant and pain reliever. They undertook a small pilot trial where teens (average age: 14) were started on 200 mg per day of SAMe, increasing the dose up to 1,400 mg if needed over the two-month study. The results were published in the journal *Alternative Therapies in*

Health and Medicine in 2013. The teens took an average of 1,400 mg per day and reported an improvement in pain. SAMe was well tolerated and no adverse effects were noted. This was an interesting study not only because SAMe has not been well studied in adolescents but also because it has not been studied in abdominal pain—intriguing!

The bulk of SAMe is produced in the liver where it has many important roles, including the synthesis of the powerful antioxidant glutathione. Glutathione is critically important for eliminating toxins from the body, preventing damage to our DNA, and keeping our mitochrondrial powerhouses functioning properly. If the liver is stressed, whether from alcohol, drugs, environmental toxins, or poor diet, SAMe levels fall and so does glutathione, making it more difficult for the liver to do its job. It is a vicious cycle. Early research suggests SAMe may help slow the progression of liver disease. And while we need clinical trials to truly understand the role SAMe might play in liver health, it can certainly be considered when thinking about an integrative treatment strategy.

WHO MIGHT BENEFIT FROM SUPPLEMENTING: Those with arthritis, fibromyalgia, chronic pain, and/or depression might benefit from SAMe supplements. If you have more severe depression, please work with a trusted health-care professional to determine whether SAMe may be appropriate for you.

HOW MUCH SHOULD YOU TAKE: Always start low and go slow. I have patients take 200 mg twice a day, early in the morning and in the afternoon, for three or four days and then increase by 200 mg every three days until they are at 1,000 to 1,200 mg per day. People over the age of 65 often get relief with just 400 to 600 mg per day.

SUPPLEMENT CONSIDERATIONS: SAMe must be enteric-coated to prevent its destruction by stomach acid. Don't cut your SAMe pills in half or you'll destroy the coating. It can be expensive, but it is effective. It's best to take SAMe on an empty stomach, but if it causes stomach upset, take it with food. SAMe works closely with folate and vitamins B2, B6, and B12 and a deficiency in any of these vitamins can lower SAMe levels, making us more vulnerable to impaired cognition, depressed mood, and poor sleep. This is why it is very important to take SAMe along with your multivitamin or B-complex to ensure it has the right partners to do its job.

DRUG INTERACTIONS: Do not take SAMe if you are taking prescription antidepressant medications, as it might bring about a rare condition called serotonin syndrome, in which too much serotonin builds up in the brain. Serotonin syndrome is less likely but could also occur if you take SAMe with tramadol (Ultram), meperidine (Demerol), or pentazocine (Talwin), and an even rarer risk if you take it with dextromethorphan (cough syrups, such as Robitussin DM). Do not take SAMe with levodopa, a drug used to treat Parkinson's disease.

SAFETY: SAMe is actually quite well tolerated in clinical trials. I've had hundreds of patients who've taken it over the years with good results and few problems. SAMe can be stimulating, which is one reason why I think many people who are in pain, depressed, and tired find that it works so well for them. But antidepressants that have stimulating effects should not be used in people with bipolar depression, on the rare chance it could trigger a manic episode. Although SAMe has been used to treat certain conditions during pregnancy, you should always talk to your health-care provider before taking it if you are pregnant or breastfeeding.

SAMe has not been well studied in children under the age of 12, though the study at UC, San Diego found it was well tolerated in 14-year-olds.

A PERSONALIZED APPROACH TO SUPPLEMENTS

So, there you have it: a few of my favorite nutraceuticals. As I said at the beginning of this chapter, I selected those that I use often and that I thought could be important to a broad range of people. Alpha-lipoic acid, particularly with acetyl-l-carnitine, may give us a healthy edge when it comes to aging. And with the growing number of people with diabetes, the fact that alpha-lipoic acid can treat, and I believe help prevent, diabetic neuropathy makes it a powerful tool.

Choline could have easily been included in the vitamin chapter since it must be consumed in our diet and has a recommended daily allowance. Yet most people have never even heard of it! The evidence that adequate amounts consumed during pregnancy and infancy can enhance our children's resiliency and tolerance to stress seems like a message that should be more loudly discussed. And the fact that most pregnant women aren't getting enough or that it's not in most prenatal vitamins is concerning. Choline helps reduce the risk of fatty liver, a condition we're seeing in younger and younger people that can cause fatigue, nausea, confusion, trouble concentrating, and eventually, cirrhosis.

Our mitochondria are crucial for providing fuel for our cells and there are many scientists who believe that when they are damaged, the diseases associated with aging occur. We make less CoQ10 as we age, while cardiovascular and neurological diseases increase. Studies show that CoQ10 helps maintain the health of our arteries, lowers blood pressure, and improves the pumping action of our heart. It can prevent migraine headaches and may offer additional support to the aging brain.

Osteoarthritis is extremely common, especially as we get older, and it can be debilitating. I trained for many years in the Korean martial art Tae Kwon Do. For roughly five of those years, I was training 18 hours every week. I ended up with a hip replacement at the age of 46. I have no regrets, but given what I know now, I certainly would have taken glucosamine and chondroitin during those years of training and beyond. I tell anyone who does repetitive sports to consider supplementation, as well as recommend it to my patients with arthritis. Why wouldn't you take something that can slow the progression of the disease, preserving your joints, reducing your need for pain medication, and delaying the need for surgery?

We live in a world of light. We light up the day and the night. We're on our laptops and smartphones until late at night, the television playing in the background. Just about everything about 21st-century life delays and diminishes our production of melatonin. Melatonin, the ancient hormone that has maintained our internal clock since the beginning of time, may be more important to our health than we ever realized. Not only can it help us sleep, it can improve mood, ease pain, eliminate heartburn, and possibly even protect our cells from cancer. I take it every single evening.

I don't think there's anyone in the U.S. that hasn't heard that eating fish is good for you. I was raised on catfish, perch, and blue gill. And yet, one-third of Americans never eat any seafood. You could get some of those precious omega-3s from beef if the cows spent their lives in grassy pastures. But most of the beef we eat is grain-fed and high in omega-6. Omega-3-rich eggs can be a good source of DHA but many people still think the yolks are bad for you, opting for the egg white spinach omelet. The yolk is where you'll find the DHA, as well as choline and a whole host of other nutrients! During pregnancy babies must have adequate amounts of DHA for their brain and eyes to develop properly, and yet many pregnant women avoid fish because of mercury concerns and many prenatal supplements don't contain it. We need EPA and DHA to dial back the inflammation that is driving so much chronic disease. You either need to eat foods rich in EPA and DHA or you need to consider taking supplements.

The American diet is woefully lacking in probiotic rich, fermented foods. My mother loved sauerkraut; I hated it. My father grew up drinking buttermilk. The only time I ever had it was when my mom was making pancakes. I admit I didn't learn much about the human microbiome during my medical training. I certainly never knew that an imbalance in these microorganisms could cause intestinal hyperpermeability and systemic inflammation, or that being born by C-section could lead to so many long-term health problems. I've prescribed my share of antibiotics and I like to think I did so only when necessary. But never did I think that I could be contributing to obesity, asthma, or autoimmune disease. I never prescribe antibiotics anymore without also recommending months of probiotics. I encourage all pregnant patients and friends to take probiotics during the last six weeks of pregnancy and to give it to their baby if born by C-section or if the baby is at high risk for allergies or eczema. And I'm happy to report that today, my family avidly consumes full-fat, probiotic-rich Greek yogurt four or five days every week. And we keep a bottle of probiotics in the refrigerator, just in case.

And finally, there is SAMe. Our body can make this important compound if given the proper nutrition and the liver is not overtaxed. However, as I mentioned previously, many Americans are deficient in the B-vitamins that are necessary for the synthesis of SAMe and our liver has to process more toxins than ever before. SAMe can be a powerful remedy for those living with chronic pain and/or depression. I've listened to the many patients who've found it life changing, and have heard similar reports from many of my integrative colleagues.

I know that some of you will wish I'd discussed your favorite supplement or one that you've been hearing about lately on the news. If I didn't write about a particular nutraceutical, it doesn't mean that it's not beneficial or I don't think it works. It's just that I had to select a small handful and these were the ones I really wanted to share.

Chapter 6

Supplements for Common Ailments

For most people, taking a multivitamin-mineral supplement should fill in many of the potential gaps that exist in their diets. Many will also benefit from additional vitamin D, and possibly magnesium, probiotics, and omega-3 fatty acids if they don't regularly eat seafood. For those living with a specific medical condition or in a particular life stage (pregnant, elder years, etc.), it's important to consider additional supplements to support overall health.

As someone who cared for pregnant women for many years, I am deeply distraught knowing that many do not get the nutrients they need to optimize their baby's health. And what mother, or father, doesn't want to start a child off with the very best possible health? While folate remains vitally important, so are vitamins B7 (biotin), B12, and D, as well as calcium, choline, iodine, iron, and omega-3 fatty acids. They are all important for your health, and the health of your little one.

If you're breastfeeding, congratulations! However, your infant is relying solely upon you for the first six months of his or her life. We can't give what we don't have, which is why you need to give your baby 400 IU each day of vitamin D. If he or she was born by C-section you might want to consider giving your child probiotics for the first 6 to 12 months of his or her life (talk to your health-care provider). You need to continue taking your prenatal, as well as making sure you are getting plenty of choline and omega-3 fatty acids.

Children need to make sure they are getting healthy nutrition. But many may not be. A basic children's multivitamin-mineral supplement, along with some omega-3 fatty acids, might be a very good idea. Kids often get sick and take antibiotics. If that's the case, don't forget the probiotics.

Teenagers often seem invincible but we know they aren't. When I was a teen, we had two beverage choices: milk or water. Today, most teens drink lots of soda pop and energy drinks. Where are they getting their calcium and vitamin D? Now is the time for them to build strong bones. We often think of calcium for the girls, but boys' bones are bigger and their need for calcium is great. They also need plenty of zinc as they move through puberty, but most don't get enough. Teenage girls may become low in iron because of the heavy, irregular periods that often characterize puberty. Iron deficiency anemia can slow down a teen girl both physically and mentally. And while parents never like to think their teenage daughter may be sexually active, getting her started on 200 to 400 mcg of folate in a basic multivitamin will offer her baby protection should she get pregnant. What I'm trying to say is that children and teens often benefit from supplements in places where the diet comes up lacking.

As we age, our needs change and some of our body's nutrient "machinery" works less efficiently. As our skin thins with age, it becomes more difficult to synthesize vitamin D. When our vitamin D levels fall too low, we begin to feel pain in our lower back as well as our hips and legs. Our muscles become weaker, and our bones are more likely to fracture. We make less CoQ10, which is vitally important to our mitochondria, the powerhouses of our cells. This nutrient helps maintain the health of blood vessels, reducing the risk of atherosclerosis. It also keeps our blood pressure from climbing and supports the pumping action of our heart. As stomach acid declines, it is harder to absorb B12 from our food. Low B12 can leave us feeling fatigued and causes our memory to become less sharp. We can become depressed. Many of us develop marginal deficiencies in riboflavin, which is necessary for activating B6 and assisting folate in the conversion of homocysteine to methionine. Elevated levels of homocysteine are associated with an increased risk for heart disease, stroke, and peripheral vascular disease—all conditions we are vulnerable to with age. As we get older, many of us will end up taking prescription medications, which can further deplete our nutrients. Supplements can be an incredibly important, and often an essential tool, for healthy aging.

Many medical conditions can make us more vulnerable for certain nutrient deficiencies. Ensuring that we are getting enough of the right vitamins and minerals and key nutraceuticals may help slow the progression of our diabetes or heart disease as well as improve our quality of life. If taking glucosamine and chondroitin can delay a knee replacement, helping maintain the connective tissue around the joint and easing pain, what a gift! If taking fish oil reduces inflammation in the body, think about what the long-term benefits might be. Why not try melatonin for six to eight weeks to alleviate GERD before signing up for possibly years of taking a proton-pump inhibitor that may have numerous adverse effects?

I will repeat myself once again, because it bears repeating: I believe that the foundation of good health is healthy, fresh, wholesome food, regular physical activity, nourishing and restful sleep, a strong social network, and limited exposure to toxins, including not smoking. I believe that a health-care practitioner you can partner with on your journey is priceless and worth investing some of your time and energy into finding. I do not believe vitamins, minerals, and other supplements are magic pills. However, I do believe that they can be used strategically and wisely to improve our health.

Following is a chart of vitamins, minerals, and nutraceuticals that I have created based upon the earlier chapters in this book. This list does NOT mean that you should take all of them, but rather these are the supplements you might want to investigate further given your unique health situation. If you are taking prescription or over-the-counter medications, use this chart in conjunction with the chart found in Appendix 4, "Drug-Nutrient Depletions and Interactions." I encourage you to talk with a qualified health-care professional that is familiar with the use of dietary supplements before taking high doses of any supplement, especially to treat any particular medical condition. If you are interested in using botanical or herbal supplements to address some of these conditions, I encourage you to read my books *Healthy at Home* and the *National Geographic Guide to Medicinal Herbs.*

CONDITION/CONCERN OR SPECIAL CONSIDERATION

Supplements to Investigate

Condition/Concern	Supplements	Suggested Combinations
ADHD	Calcium, iodine, iron, magnesium, melatonin, vitamin B5 (pantothenic acid), omega-3 fatty acids	Consider taking a high-quality multivitamin-mineral and melatonin if having difficulty sleeping.
Alcoholism/regular alcohol consumption	Vitamin A, all B-vitamins (esp. B1, B2, B3, B6), vitamin K, choline, magnesium, zinc	Consider taking a high-quality multivitamin-mineral with emphasis on higher levels of B-vitamins.

Condition/Concern	Supplements	Suggested Combinations
Anemia	Vitamins A, B2 (riboflavin), B6 (pyridoxine), B9 (folate), B12 (cobalamin); iron, zinc	If taking iron supplements, consider taking with vitamins A, B2 (riboflavin), and C.
Anxiety, depression	Vitamins B6 (pyridoxine), B9 (folate), B12 (cobalamin), and D; omega-3 fatty acids, calcium choline, magnesium, melatonin, SAMe	Consider taking a multivitamin-mineral with higher levels of B-vitamins; look for those with methylfolate, methylcobalamin, and P5P to ensure optimal benefit. Consider taking melatonin if difficulty sleeping. Magnesium is naturally calming. SAMe *may* be appropriate.
Arthritis	SAMe, glucosamine with chondroitin, vitamins B6 (pyridoxine), C and D; niacin; selenium, magnesium, zinc, omega-3 fatty acids	Strongly consider taking glucosamine and chondroitin long term, omega-3 fatty acids to lower inflammation, and possibly SAMe for pain.
Brain health	Vitamins B1 (thiamine), B6 (pyridoxine), B12 (cobalamin), E, folate, niacin; magnesium, alpha-lipoic acid, acetyl-l-carnitine, DHA, CoQ10, omega-3 fatty acids, iodine, iron, choline, probiotics	Consider taking a multivitamin-mineral with higher levels of B-vitamins; look for those with methylfolate, methylcobalamin, and P5P to ensure optimal benefit. Omega-3 fatty acids are foundational. Consider taking alpha-lipoic acid and acetyl-l-carnitine.
Breast health	Vitamin B6 (pyridoxine), calcium, iodine, melatonin	Vitamin B6 and calcium reduce tenderness associated with menses.
Cancer and cancer prevention	Niacin, folate, vitamins B6 (pyridoxine), B12 (cobalamin), C, D, E, K; iodine, selenium, zinc, choline, melatonin, omega-3 fatty acids	You should *always* talk to your health-care provider before taking supplements, if you are undergoing cancer treatment.
Celiac disease	Vitamins B2 (riboflavin), B3 (niacin), B6 (pyridoxine), B9 (folate), B12 (cobalamin) and D, calcium, magnesium, zinc, probiotics	Take a multivitamin-mineral. Check binders and fillers for gluten. Ensure probiotics are gluten free.
Cholesterol, high	Niacin, pantothenic acid, chromium, omega-3 fatty acids, choline	Omega-3 fatty acids lower triglycerides. Do not use high-dose niacin without supervision. Choline should be considered. Investigate red yeast rice and phytosterols (not discussed in this book).

Condition/Concern	Supplements	Suggested Combinations
Constipation	Vitamin B1 (thiamine), magnesium, melatonin, probiotics, iodine	Magnesium is natural laxative. Use calcium citrate if taking calcium supplements. Probiotics and melatonin effective if IBS.
Cystic fibrosis	Vitamins A, D, E, and K; calcium, iron, zinc, omega-3 fatty acids, pancreatic enzymes	Take high-quality multivitamin-mineral. Keep vitamin D level >30 ng/mL. Do not take >150 mcg potassium iodide in supplement.
Diabetes	Vitamins B1 (thiamine), B6 (pyridoxine), B7 (biotin), B12 (cobalamin), C, D, and K; calcium, choline, chromium, iodine, magnesium, zinc, melatonin, alpha-lipoic acid	Take a high-quality multivitamin-mineral. Take vitamin B12 if on metformin. Strongly consider supplementing with thiamine and magnesium. Consider taking alpha-lipoic acid to protect nerves. Choline to reduce risk of fatty liver disease.
Diarrhea	Melatonin, probiotics, zinc	Take melatonin if diarrhea is due to IBS. Probiotics no matter the cause of diarrhea. If persistent diarrhea, consider taking 15–25 mg of zinc per day, as well as a multivitamin-mineral. Cut back on magnesium and vitamin C, which can loosen stools.
Ethnicity: African American, Hispanic	May be at higher risk for deficiencies in iron, vitamins B1 (thiamine), B3 (niacin), B6 (pyridoxine) and D; magnesium and omega-3 fatty acids	African Americans more likely to be deficient in iron, and vitamins B1, B6, and D. Hispanics more likely to be deficient in niacin, magnesium, and folate.
European	At higher risk for hemochromatosis, causing iron buildup	
Eye health	Vitamins A, B6 (pyridoxine), B7 (biotin), B9 (folate), B12 (cobalamin) and C; zinc, omega-3 fatty acids (DHA)	Take DHA for dry eyes, vitamin A and zinc if difficulty seeing in dim light. Talk to eye doctor about Ocu-Vite if you have age-related macular degeneration. Do not supplement with B12 if you have Leber's disease.
Fibrocystic breast disease	Vitamin E, iodine	Some women report benefit with high-dose vitamin E but there is little evidence to support its use.
Fibromyalgia	Iodine, melatonin, SAMe, vitamin D	Consider taking SAMe and/or melatonin. Maintain vitamin D level at >30 ng/mL.

Condition/Concern	Supplements	Suggested Combinations
Gout	Vitamin C	Taking 500 mg twice daily enhances excretion of uric acid.
Hemochromatosis	Chromium	Avoid excess vitamin C and do not take supplemental iron. Chromium absorption impaired, which may increase risk for diabetes, consider supplement.
Heart health	Vitamins B1 (thiamine), B3 (niacin), B6 (pyridoxine), B9 (folate), B12 (cobalamin), D, E, and K; choline, magnesium, omega-3 fatty acids, CoQ10	Research these supplements carefully to determine which are best for your particular heart concern.
Heartburn/GERD	Calcium, melatonin	Consider a trial of melatonin for heartburn. Calcium is effective for occasional relief.
Immune support	Vitamins A, C, D and all B-vitamins; zinc, melatonin, iodine, iron, selenium, omega-3 fatty acids, probiotics	Research these supplements carefully to find which are most appropriate for your situation. If you've taken many antibiotics, strongly consider probiotics.
Inflammatory bowel disease (Crohn's, ulcerative colitis)	Vitamins A, B6 (pyridoxine), B9 (folate), B12 (cobalamin), D, E, and K; chromium, iron, magnesium, zinc, omega-3 fatty acids, probiotics	Nutrient deficiency is common and lab testing often necessary. A multivitamin-mineral, probiotics, and omega-3 fatty acids are foundational. Investigate turmeric, not discussed in this book.
Irritable bowel syndrome (IBS)	Melatonin, probiotics, vitamin B6 (pyridoxine), calcium, magnesium, enteric-coated peppermint oil	Probiotics are a must. Enteric-coated peppermint oil has good evidence. Consider taking melatonin. Look under "Diarrhea" and "Constipation" for specifics.
Kidney stones	Vitamins B6 (pyridoxine), and C; calcium citrate and magnesium	These supplements most useful for preventing calcium oxalate stones. Take vitamin C for uric acid kidney stones.
Kidney disease	Vitamins B1 (thiamine), B6 (pyridoxine), C; iron, selenium, zinc	Speak with your health-care provider about what supplements may be important for you.
Lifestyle: Adolescent boys and adult men under 50	Vitamin D, magnesium, and zinc. Calcium and thiamine, especially during growth spurt	Ensure adequate calcium, zinc, and vitamin D in adolescent boys. Adult men should be cautious with calcium supplements until its relationship with prostate cancer is better understood.

Condition/Concern	Supplements	Suggested Combinations
Lifestyle: Adolescent girl or menstruating adult woman, not pregnant or breastfeeding	Vitamins B1 (thiamine), B2 (riboflavin), B6 (pyridoxine), B9 (folate), and D; calcium, magnesium, iron. Thiamine during growth spurt.	Strongly consider taking a multi-vitamin-mineral with iron and 400 mcg per day of methylfolate. Ensure adequate calcium and vitamin D. Heavy menstruation can be a sign of low vitamin K and lead to iron deficiency.
Lifestyle: Athlete	Vitamins B1 (thiamine), B2 (riboflavin), and D; chromium, iron, omega-3 fatty acids	Ensure adequate B-vitamins. Female athletes should maintain adequate calcium and vitamin D for bone health.
Lifestyle: Blood donor	Iron, vitamin C	If you donate regularly, you need iron supplementation.
Lifestyle: Breastfeeding	Vitamins A, C, D, K and all B-vitamins; calcium, choline, iodine, iron, magnesium, zinc, and omega-3 fatty acids.	Take prenatal vitamins while breastfeeding. Consider taking additional calcium and vitamin D. Aim for 550 mg of choline and 200–500 mg per day of DHA.
Lifestyle: Child	Multivitamin with D, iron, calcium, choline, zinc, probiotics	Work with an integrative pediatrician or dietitian to determine your child's needs.
Lifestyle: Infants	Probiotics, vitamin D, iron, choline, omega-3 fatty acids (DHA)	Consider probiotics if born premature, by C-section, or at high risk for allergies. Give 400 IU per day vitamin D if breastfed.
Lifestyle: Over 50, male	Multivitamin-mineral, vitamins B12 (cobalamin), and D; magnesium, choline, omega-3 fatty acids, alpha-lipoic acid, acetyl-l-carnitine	Do not supplement with iron unless specifically told to. Maintain vitamin D level at >30 ng/mL. Take a multivitamin-mineral with higher B12.
Lifestyle: Perimenopausal or post-menopausal woman (one year without menstruation)	Multivitamin-mineral, vitamins B6 (pyridoxine), B12 (cobalamin), D, and K; calcium, magnesium, choline, melatonin, zinc, omega-3 fatty acids, alpha-lipoic acid, acetyl-l-carnitine	Take a multivitamin-mineral with higher B12. Ensure adequate calcium, magnesium, vitamin K, and zinc. Maintain vitamin D level at >30 ng/mL. Consider taking melatonin. No iron once postmenopausal unless specifically told to take it.
Lifestyle: Pregnant	Prenatal multivitamin and mineral; vitamins B1 (thiamine), B6 (pyridoxine), B7 (biotin), B9 (folate) and D; calcium, choline, iodine, iron, magnesium, omega-3 fatty acids (esp. DHA), selenium, zinc	Ensure prenatal includes (or supplement): 150–250 mcg of iodine, 200 mg DHA, 300–500 mg choline, 300 mcg biotin, and 400 mcg methylfolate. Maintain vitamin D level at >30 ng/mL.

Condition/Concern	Supplements	Suggested Combinations
Lifestyle: Smoking	Vitamins B7 (biotin), C, and E	Avoid beta-carotene supplements or do not exceed 2,500 IU per day. Consider taking 250 mg twice daily of vitamin C.
Lifestyle: Stress (emotional, mental)	All B-vitamins, vitamin C; chromium, omega-3 fatty acids, probiotics, melatonin	Consider taking a multivitamin-mineral with higher levels B-vitamins, additional vitamin C, and omega-3 fatty acids.
Lifestyle: Vegans and vegetarians	Vitamins B6 (pyridoxine), B12 (cobalamin), D2, K; choline, iodine, iron, zinc, omega-3 fatty acids	Take a multivitamin-mineral specific for vegans or vegetarians that includes B12. Take non-marine omega-3 fatty acids.
Liver support	Vitamins B1 (thiamine), B6 (pyridoxine), B9 (folate), B12 (cobalamin), and E; alpha-lipoic acid, choline, SAMe, selenium	Take a multivitamin with B--vitamins. Consider taking choline for fatty liver disease, SAMe may be helpful. Talk to health-care provider if you have severe liver disease.
Low energy, fatigue	Vitamins B5 (pantothenic acid), B6 (pyridoxine), B7 (biotin), B9 (folate), B12 (cobalamin), C and D; calcium, iodine, iron, magnesium, melatonin, SAMe	There are many underlying causes for fatigue and low energy. Ensure you are properly evaluated.
Male fertility	CoQ10, potassium, selenium, zinc, vitamins C and E	These supplements may be beneficial as part of an integrative strategy.
Migraines	Magnesium, melatonin, CoQ10, vitamin B2 (riboflavin)	The Canadian Headache Society gives magnesium citrate, riboflavin, and CoQ10 a "strongly recommend" for the prevention of migraines.
Morning sickness	Vitamins B1 (thiamine), B6 (pyridoxine)	The American College of Obstetrics and Gynecology considers vitamin B6 a first-line treatment for nausea and vomiting caused by pregnancy. If you have prolonged vomiting, thiamine may become an issue.
Multiple sclerosis	Vitamins B6 (pyridoxine), B7 (biotin), B12 (cobalamin) and D; calcium and omega-3 fatty acids	Ensure vitamin D levels >30 ng/mL. Consider taking biotin and high-dose omega-3 fatty acids.
Muscle tension, aches, weakness	Vitamins B1 (thiamine), D and E; CoQ10, calcium, iron, magnesium, SAMe	Determine what is causing your muscle aches and/or weakness, to use supplements most effectively.

Condition/Concern	Supplements	Suggested Combinations
Obesity	Probiotics, iodine, calcium, chromium, vitamins B1 (thiamine), B6 (pyridoxine), and D.	Obesity can lead to a number of nutrient deficiencies; these are some of the most common. Read their respective sections to learn more.
Oral health	Vitamins B6 (pyridoxine), B9 (folate), B12 (cobalamin), C, D and K; calcium, zinc, CoQ10, omega-3 fatty acids, probiotics	All of these nutrients are important for reducing oral inflammation, preserving taste, and maintaining healthy teeth.
Osteoporosis/low bone density	Vitamins B12 (cobalamin), D, and K; calcium, magnesium, potassium, zinc, and other trace minerals.	Maintain vitamin D level at >30 ng/mL. Ensure adequate calcium, magnesium, zinc, vitamin K, and trace minerals.
Premenstrual syndrome (PMS)	Vitamin B6 (pyridoxine), calcium, magnesium	Calcium and B6 shown to be beneficial for PMS. Magnesium helpful for menstrual cramps.
Respiratory health: allergies, asthma, bronchitis, cold/cough	Vitamins A, C, and D; magnesium, zinc, omega-3 fatty acids, probiotics	Supplement needs will vary depending upon your underlying health concern.
Restless leg syndrome	Iron	Talk to your health-care provider about the use of iron.
Sickle-cell anemia	Zinc, vitamins B9 (folate) and D	Take zinc to reduce infection. Use probiotics if taking frequent antibiotics. Folate supplements often needed.
Sleep	Melatonin, magnesium, vitamin B6 (pyridoxine)	B-vitamins are necessary for synthesizing melatonin. Consider taking melatonin if having trouble falling asleep. Magnesium is calming before bedtime.
Vaginal dryness	Vitamin E suppositories, probiotics	Vitamin E suppositories can be very soothing. Probiotics to maintain vaginal pH.
Wound healing	Vitamins B5 (pantothenic acid) and C; zinc, omega-3 fatty acids	Vitamin C and zinc are vitally important in the healing of wounds. Topical zinc and B5 both used to mend wounds.

Chapter 7

Making Sense of Health Information

"Multivitamins don't work."

"Fish oil is good."

"Fish oil is bad."

"Take your vitamin D."

Seems like the news is full of commentary about nutritional supplements these days. You've likely heard all of these broad pronouncements, or others like them, but they're not at all helpful for deciding what nutritional supplements *you* might need. Flip-flops in the news are commonplace, and it can make it hard to figure out what is best for you and your family. Remember when we were told butter was bad? Everyone started eating margarine. Whoops! Margarine contains trans fats, which are much worse for you than saturated fat ever was. Eggs are good. No, eggs are bad. Wait—eggs really *are* good for you. No wonder so many people are confused about foods and supplements!

I hope that this book has provided a firm foundation of knowledge about nutritional supplements. But there will always be another headline, another new miracle pill offered. To be a savvy consumer of health information, particularly when it comes to supplements, you have to understand a few things about health news, nutritional research, physicians, the laws that regulate dietary supplements, and the supplement companies themselves. The more you know, the easier it will be to tune out the noise and focus on the information that will benefit you the most. Here are some tools for navigating through the onslaught of media and marketing surrounding supplements these days.

Do you have a medical condition? Are you taking prescription medications? Finding a health-care practitioner to partner with isn't always easy. As a physician, I was extremely well trained in the diagnosis and treatment of disease. Physicians, like other professionals, practice what we know. When it comes to counseling a patient on nutrition or the use of herbal medicines or dietary supplements, we are at a profound disadvantage. As someone who ran the postgraduate fellowship program for physicians at the University of Arizona Center for Integrative Medicine for many years, I can tell you firsthand that doctors do *not* know how to counsel patients on these topics. Medical schools and residency programs are trying to step up their teaching in these areas but unfortunately, the chances are high that your doctor or nurse practitioner is not familiar with which supplements interact with a particular drug or if the medication you are taking is depleting you of a particular nutrient.

Many Americans, especially those over the age of 50, take multiple medications. A common combination I see is someone taking a proton pump inhibitor (PPI), such as Prilosec or Nexium, for their heartburn/acid reflux, metformin for their diabetes, and an ACE inhibitor for their blood pressure. The person comes to my office feeling tired and depressed, and is catching every cold going around the office. I begin to think about the possibility of nutritional deficiencies.

Let's start with the PPIs. The FDA has mandated a warning that using these drugs over the long term (more than one year) may increase the risk of fractures of the hip, wrist, and spine due in part to poor absorption of calcium. Long-term use of PPIs also depletes the body of magnesium (increasing the risk for seizures and heart arrhythmia), iron (needed to transport oxygen around the body), and vitamin B12 (a nutrient that is critically important for the brain and nervous system). PPIs also increase the risk for pneumonia and infection with the bacterium *Clostridium difficile,* which can be very difficult to treat—it's the bug that made my father so ill, as I described early in this book. While metformin is a very effective drug for diabetes, the longer you take it, the greater the chance you will become depleted in vitamin B12. Vitamin B12 deficiency can cause tingling in the hands and feet, as well as depression, confusion, memory loss, dementia, and difficulty maintaining balance. Finally, ACE inhibitors deplete both zinc and magnesium. Low magnesium is associated with metabolic syndrome, type 2 diabetes, heart disease, sudden cardiac death, osteoporosis, migraines, and asthma. Zinc is vitally important for the proper function of immune system. Yet virtually no one is being counseled by their physician about the need to increase their dietary intake of foods rich in these nutrients or to take supplements to prevent deficiencies. Could nutrient depletion explain why my 70-year-old patient who has been on these medications for many years is now depressed and has osteoporosis, diminished memory, and a sluggish immune response? Or is it simply all due to "old age?" I guarantee you that many patients just end up being placed on more drugs to treat these symptoms instead of getting at the root of what is causing them.

It's important that you are educated about and aware of how your nutrition, lifestyle, and medications impact your health. You must be your own health advocate. I will go into more specifics about potential interactions between medications, nutrients, and dietary supplements later in the book, but now I would like to give some practical advice on how to weather the information storm.

BREAKING NEWS! WHAT TO MAKE OF THAT STORY ON TV

Not long ago, I was watching television with my husband, Jim, and the health reporter began to talk about a study of elderly Japanese people and baby aspirin: The research showed that taking one baby aspirin a day did not reduce their risk of having a heart attack or stroke, or from dying from a heart attack. "Aren't there studies that show baby aspirin reduces the risk for dying of a heart attack?" Jim asked. "Seems like Japanese people do a lot of things differently than Americans. They eat more fish and seaweed and less red meat. And they're generally much thinner than we are. So, do these results apply to someone like me?" Jim knows how to ask the right questions when he hears about a supplement or medication being "good" or "bad" for this reason or that.

There are some key questions to consider when evaluating research. Each will help you uncover the information you need to know to decide whether this is a study to pay attention to, because it can help you make better health decisions for you and your family, or whether it's one that simply doesn't have much value for you.

QUESTION 1: Do the findings contradict other studies, or do other studies support these findings?
In the early 1990s, researchers in Cuba isolated a component of sugarcane wax called policosanol and produced a supplement

from it. Then these researchers conducted studies and found that it dramatically lowered cholesterol. Within just a few years, policosanol was approved as a cholesterol-lowering drug in many Caribbean and South American countries. However, when independent research teams at Rush University, the University of Kansas, McGill University in Montreal, and in Italy conducted similar trials using policosanol, not a single one found any beneficial effect on cholesterol, at any dose.

Studies from *independent research teams* are needed to confirm findings. This is why scientists publish their research methods and statistical analyses in peer-reviewed journals. This allows other researchers to critique the study, as well as attempt to duplicate the findings. Sometimes, research is blatantly falsified but fortunately, that is not common. More often, the study just wasn't methodologically rigorous. Peer-reviewed journals can get it wrong. Don't be too quick to believe a study that is an outlier, whether positive or negative. *The findings of a single study seldom prove or disprove anything.*

QUESTION 2: Why is this news?

The goal of health reporting is primarily to gain viewers' attention and keep them tuned in. It is *really* important to realize that when one more study comes out and says pretty much the same thing as the last 10 studies, the study probably isn't going to make the evening news. If a research study offers the opportunity for a shocking headline, you'll find it showing up in all sorts of news outlets. But in the context of your health, the new research might not be that significant.

A while back, there were reports that organic produce was no more nutritious than conventionally grown produce. The take-home message seemed to be "expensive organic foods aren't any better for you." Assuming for the moment that this study was sound, and backed by other studies, think about why most people buy organics and believe they are "better": not because they have more nutrients than nonorganic produce but because they are lower in pesticides, which have been associated with numerous risks to human and environmental health. In other words, it might not matter to you that the organic orange you purchased wasn't higher in vitamin C than the nonorganic. You buy organic to avoid the pesticides. And just for the record, a 2014 *British Journal of Nutrition* article concluded after reviewing 343 scientific papers that organic produce *does* have higher concentrations of important antioxidants, lower concentrations of the toxic metal cadmium, and a lower incidence of pesticide residues when compared to nonorganic crops.

When it comes to real-world situations that a clinician like me or an individual like you faces, researchers aren't always in touch with what goes on outside of their labs. In December 2013, a study in the *Annals of Internal Medicine* made a lot of headlines because researchers found that high-dose multivitamins (six pills per day) did not prevent a second heart attack in patients with heart disease. I'm not saying that the research wasn't useful; however, is that really why most people take a multivitamin? Because they believe it will keep them from having another heart attack? And do most people take six multivitamins a day? And is that study any reason to conclude that multivitamins "don't work?" Most people take multivitamins primarily to prevent nutrient gaps in their diet.

QUESTION 3: Does the story or health claim pass the common-sense test?

If your instincts say, "That can't be right," listen to them. Be skeptical, listen to your gut, and gather more information before drawing any firm conclusions. There's a lot of flaky information out there. Some manufacturers make wild claims for their products. If you hear promises that a supplement will cure cancer, lupus, or another complex condition, feel free to roll your eyes. The supplement might *help* with the condition, but if it could actually *cure* it, you would have heard about it on the nightly news, from the CDC or the National Institutes of Health. Breakthrough news about a supplement's "showing promise" for treating a disease is the kind of good news that *is* worthy of your attention if you or someone you know has the disease. But remember, science is cumulative; it takes time to figure out what works and what doesn't.

QUESTION 4: Was the study a meta-analysis of existing studies?

A meta-analysis is a statistical technique for looking at data from numerous studies. These analyses are very useful for assessing large amounts of research for their rigor and potential bias. How many of the studies were sponsored by a drug or supplement company? How many of the studies were randomized and double-blinded? Randomized studies assign participants to the placebo group or the supplement or drug group randomly, to prevent bias from affecting the research. In double-blind studies, neither the patients nor the researchers know who is taking the supplement or drug and who is taking the placebo—an inert sugar pill made to look just like the real thing. Keeping everyone in the dark about which pills contain active ingredients and which don't prevents the beliefs of the researcher or patient from influencing the results. Double-blind studies work well for drugs and many dietary supplements; however, they are not very suitable for nutrition (food) studies or modalities, such as acupuncture or massage.

There are other questions to ask, too. How were the results calculated and reported? Of course, meta-analyses can get it wrong by not including all studies (both published and unpublished), not adequately looking for bias, or not using the appropriate statistical methods. While meta-analyses can be helpful for making general recommendations about a treatment, they can fall short when it comes down to what is best for an *individual*. Your own personal and family history, diet, lifestyle, and preferences must be considered when making any decision regarding the use of a particular drug or supplement.

QUESTION 5: How similar to me are the participants in the study?

My husband, Jim, immediately knew that the study evaluating the effect of baby aspirin and elder Japanese might not apply to him, any more than a 55-year-old African-American woman with diabetes, living in Detroit, could readily draw conclusions from a study on 30- to 55-year-old male doctors living in California. It's important to know that to participate in a research study, there is a relatively short inclusion list and a rather long *exclusion* list. One of my close friends and colleagues was conducting a government-funded trial on an herb for relieving menopausal hot flashes. Her team had to interview a couple thousand women to find 80 that fit all the criteria. I jokingly told her, "My patients are the 1,920 women that weren't eligible for your study. How much will this study really tell me about them?" The strict inclusion/exclusion criteria are very important to avoid unnecessary variables that might skew the results. But it does mean that the study group may only slightly resemble you.

So, when you are hearing about the results from a new study, ask yourself whether the population has a lifestyle similar to your own. Who was studied—men, women, children, people with a specific disease? What is the source of the report? A peer-reviewed journal article is generally more reliable because other experts scrutinize the paper for flaws or irregularities before it is published. Paying attention to these details will help you discern what studies are valid and apply to you.

QUESTION 6: What nutrient was being studied?

Knowing exactly what nutrient was being studied is important. As mentioned in Chapter 5, much of the reporting on glucosamine's effectiveness neglected to specify what form of glucosamine was used in the study, and whether it was combined with chondroitin. If you read something about the results of a clinical study that intrigue you, learn more about product that was actually used in the clinical trial. You may have to do a little research on the Internet, but it is generally worth the effort.

QUESTION 7: Was it a longitudinal study?

Longitudinal studies observe large numbers of people over a long period of time, and they are often very valuable for figuring out what you can do to support your health through lifestyle, diet, and nutritional supplements. One example of this type of study is the Framingham Heart Study that was initially formed in 1948 to understand the cause(s) of heart disease and stroke. The researchers enrolled and then evaluated more than 5,000 men and women aged 30 to 62 from around the town of Framingham, Massachusetts, every two years with laboratory tests, physical exams, and extensive interviewing. In 1971, the study enrolled the offspring of this original cohort, and in 2002, the third generation of participants, the grandchildren of the original cohort were enrolled. There is no substitute for this kind of longitudinal data. From the Framingham study, we learned that smoking cigarettes, having high blood pressure, being obese, and being depressed and socially isolated can all increase your risk of heart disease. The information collected over the past six decades has influenced medical practice and public policy, and has saved countless lives. Now that is a study to pay attention to.

Two other longitudinal studies are the Health Professionals Study that enrolled more than 51,000 male health professionals in 1986 and the Nurses' Health Study that has followed more than 238,000 nurse-participants since its inception in 1976. Questionnaires are sent every two years, while heavily detailed questionnaires are sent and collected every four years. The findings from these kinds of "mega-studies" that enroll large numbers of people and follow them over many years are extremely costly and time-consuming but are definitely worth the effort for the information they provide.

However, there are problems with these kinds of studies. For instance, you may not have much in common with a male physician or dentist or a female nurse. The nutrition aspect of some of these studies is also problematic in that they ask participants to recall what they have eaten over a period of time. I know from filling out one of these highly detailed nutrition questionnaires myself that it is very unlikely that anyone would really be able to accurately recall how much of a certain food he or she consumed during the past couple of months. And there is also a real risk of bias. I am sure many people don't want to put down that they drink four glasses of wine every day or eat doughnuts and Pop-Tarts for breakfast. So, while these studies are valuable, one has to use some discretion when interpreting the ones that attempt to correlate self-reported dietary histories to health outcomes.

QUESTION 8: What are some of the unique challenges for vitamin research?

Randomized, double-blinded, placebo-controlled trials are the gold standard for evaluating the effectiveness of drugs. They reduce the risk of bias and help to ensure reliable, reproducible results. However, to be enrolled in the study, patients must meet a number of criteria, including that they are drug naive, meaning that they have not taken or been exposed to the drug being currently studied.

Unfortunately, that is difficult if you are studying vitamin D, magnesium, or zinc. You can't be "nutrient naive" because these nutrients are present in your diet! To accurately study the effect of a vitamin or mineral on the body, you would have to measure levels of that nutrient(s) in a person's blood before the research begins and then at the midpoint and again at the end. Researchers often just use dietary recall to "guesstimate" someone's intake of particular nutrients, which can be notoriously inaccurate. And they have to control for many other variables, which often they do not. In the case of vitamin D, you would also have to account for different amounts of sun exposure, use of sunscreen, color of the skin, bodyweight, geographical location, as well as dietary intake of milk, fatty fish, and so forth. I could offer more examples of the complexities of researching nutritional supplements, but you get the point.

QUESTION 9: Who paid for the research?

It isn't just large corporations that manufacture and sell pharmaceutical drugs that have a lot to gain from research results. Money likely had a great deal of influence on the policosanol research being conducted in Cuba. Because a drug company or supplement manufacturer paid for the study doesn't mean that the results are invalid, however. It just means that you have to keep a little skepticism in your back pocket until independent research validates or negates the findings.

Unfortunately, there are few dietary supplement-sponsored studies of any real size or rigor. Because dietary supplement manufacturers can't patent their products, it is really difficult to convince them to pony up the cash required for research. Why would Company A spend $250,000 to conduct a study on its fish oil capsules when Companies B through Z sell a similar fish oil product? Most companies would rather spend their money on marketing, branding, and packaging. Pharmaceutical companies invest hundreds of millions of dollars to bring a new drug to market but then are also afforded patent protection to be able to recoup their investment and more.

This structure means that the institutions (often academic universities) that apply for, and are awarded, government research grants conduct the majority of supplement research in the U.S. These grants are highly competitive and when compared to other research, there is very little money to go around. Don't get me wrong. I am very grateful for the research that is being done! I just wish it were more carefully orchestrated. These products are in the marketplace and people take them, whether they are effective or not. I would like government grants to emphasize safety studies, at least as much as effectiveness studies. For instance, I wish there were more research into the potential for dietary supplements to interact with prescription medications, their impact on liver and kidney function, and their safety in children, pregnancy, and lactation. This information would be invaluable for both the public and health-care professionals.

The research process is also very slow. It leaves many people trying to figure things out on their own without any real help from their health-care team. Years ago, I was at a conference where an elder gentleman came up to me after my presentation on healthy aging. I had mentioned an ongoing study evaluating whether ginkgo was helpful for preventing cognitive decline. The man said to me, "Your presentation was wonderful. I learned so much! But I'd like to ask your personal opinion on something. I'm 85 years old and I just can't wait until that trial you mentioned finishes four or five years from now. I'm not asking for gospel. I'm asking for your best guess." I've had these kinds of questions from so many people: parents of children with autism, for example, or people with stage 4 cancer, early dementia, and other conditions for which there are few, if any, effective options. When scientific knowledge is limited, the "art" of medicine calls us to weigh the needs of the individual and the pros and cons of the intervention, and then make our "best guess."

QUESTION 10: Are there reputable websites for dietary supplement information?

There are a number of reliable websites to assist you in your research on nutrition and dietary supplements. I would like to tell you about five of them.

First, the website of the **Centers for Disease Control**, specifically its section that includes the results of the **National Health and Nutrition Examination Survey (NHANES)**, a program that assesses the health and nutritional status of 5,000 adults and children across the United States using both interviews and physical examinations. There is an exhaustive amount of information gathered through this program, although as I mentioned earlier, there are limits when it comes to recalling your diet or use of dietary supplements or over-the-counter medications over a year. This is why the *National Report on Biochemical Indicators of Diet and Nutrition in the U.S. Population* included under the CDC's Nutrition Report is so important. This program collects blood and urine samples to determine the adequacy of specific nutrient intake for the U.S. population. Here is a direct quote from the report: "Dietary deficiencies are well documented, and they have characteristic signs and symptoms. In addition, recent findings have determined that less than optimal biochemical levels have been associated with risks of adverse health effects. These health effects include cardiovascular disease, stroke, impaired cognitive function, cancer, eye diseases, poor bone health, and other conditions."

According to the CDC's most recent findings, approximately 10 percent of Hispanic children (aged 1–5), and 13 percent of Hispanic and 16 percent of African American women (aged 12–49) have iron deficiency. As a group, women aged 20 to 39 have borderline iodine insufficiency, while roughly 16 million Americans are low in vitamin C, 30 million Americans are deficient in vitamin B6, and 66 million Americans have insufficient levels of vitamin D. Wow! As you saw in earlier chapters of this book, these nutrient deficiencies are dangerous for your health. I find it incredulous that so many "experts" keep telling people that they can get everything they need in their diet! Clearly, we are not doing so!

In various places throughout this book, I have discussed the nutrient levels in certain foods. I gather most of this information the **United States Department of Agriculture Nutrient Database.** This database lists the nutrients for more than 8,000 foods. Just type in the name of the food you want to know about and it will display a long list of nutritional facts including calories, carbohydrates, fiber, protein, fats, vitamins, and minerals. When you want to know how your plate stacks up when it comes to nutrition, the U.S. Department of Agriculture Nutrient Database is very handy.

RX FROM DR. LOW DOG

Five Websites for Reliable Information on Nutrition

To access NHANES: http://www.cdc.gov/nchs/nhanes.htm

To access the CDC's nutrition report that includes the biochemical indicators:
http://www.cdc.gov/nutritionreport/

To access the U.S. Department of Agriculture Nutrient Database:
http://ndb.nal.usda.gov/

To access the NIH Office of Dietary Supplements: http://ods.od.nih.gov/

To access the Linus Pauling Institute: http://lpi.oregonstate.edu/

I am also a big fan of the **National Institutes of Health Office of Dietary Supplements.** They have an excellent website that includes a section called "Dietary Supplement Fact Sheets," where you can look up authoritative information on vitamins, minerals, and some nutraceuticals, and botanicals. They also have a mobile app called "My Dietary Supplements" that allows you to list all the names and types of supplements you take so you have them handy whether you are shopping or at your doctor's appointment. There is also a link to FDA warnings on supplements so that you can keep apprised of any products that have been found to have problems.

The **Linus Pauling Institute at Oregon State University** is also high on my list. It is a little gem if you are looking for scientifically accurate information about vitamins, minerals, and other nutrients. You can look things up by subject or by specific disease. For instance, if I select "High Blood Pressure," it will pull up the links for calcium, coenzyme Q10, magnesium, potassium, riboflavin, sodium chloride, and vitamins C and D. Clicking on any of these links takes me to a section that reviews all of the relevant evidence about how this particular nutrient affects blood pressure. This site is regularly updated and is highly reliable.

Armed with good, solid information about nutrition, and a sense of which health news reports speak to your own situation and which don't, you will be much better at taking charge of your own health.

WORKING WITH YOUR PHYSICIAN

The very best advice any physician could ever give you is to start making healthy lifestyle and dietary choices now rather than waiting until you have a serious medical problem. We must each take responsibility for our own health and well-being. And don't be surprised if you find yourself feeling a little awkward talking to your doctor after you start really educating yourself about your health. Here's a common scenario that I've heard on multiple occasions: A woman goes to see her physician for a checkup and mentions that she is taking vitamin D supplements and would like to have her vitamin D level checked. She explains that she would like to be sure it is over 30 ng/mL because she has read that this is the minimum level needed to protect her bones and possibly even reduce her risk of breast cancer. She's a savvy consumer of health care and has paid attention to the research. She mentions she is concerned because she lives in Wisconsin, uses sunscreen religiously to protect her skin, and has a family history of osteoporosis. But her doctor frowns and says she doesn't need to have her level tested. He tells her to that too much vitamin D can be dangerous. "Just take the recommended amount of vitamin D and you'll be fine." What should she do?

I hope that if this savvy consumer is you, you won't let your concerns be dismissed so easily. Those of us who went to medical school many years ago learned that because vitamin D is fat-soluble, it could build up in the body and cause problems. But now we know that the safety margin on vitamin D is actually quite wide. And studies overwhelmingly show that many Americans have low levels of vitamin D, especially those who live in northern climates. This doctor did not put all the information together in the proper context of *this woman's* body and *her* health. The fact is the farther away from the equator we live and the darker our skin, the more likely we are to be vitamin D deficient. Another risk factor for vitamin D deficiency is obesity, which currently affects one-third of the American population. Layer on the many medications that can increase your risk for low bone density, such as steroids, proton pump inhibitors, antipsychotics, some antidepressants, anti-seizure medications, and drugs used to treat prostate and breast cancer and you have a recipe for osteoporosis and fracture. Low vitamin D increases your risk for falls and muscle weakness, making it even more likely you may suffer a fracture. It may also increase your risk for dying from heart disease and certain cancers. In the scenario above, it is very reasonable to request having your vitamin D level checked.

Some health-care practitioners might feel a little intimidated when they realize a patient has done her homework and might know more about a particular topic than they do. I understand; I'm a doctor. It's part of our professional DNA and training. The first year after graduating medical school you do your internship, which typically involves doing morning rounds where you evaluate all the patients your team is responsible for in the hospital. It is very common for the lead or attending physician to turn to the intern and quickly throw out a question. Of course, you're expected to know the answer on the spot. With everyone watching—sometimes, including the patient—you wrack your brain to make sure you announce the right answer. There is tremendous pressure to be the smartest person in the room, and to never say, "I don't know." The culture is stressful and it's very easy to fear being wrong and feeling shamed. In fact, this high-pressure "answer the question before the buzzer rings!" makes a doctor-in-training feel very vulnerable. It can also make it difficult for physicians to admit that they don't know something.

Fortunately, more and more physicians, and other health-care practitioners, are aware that thanks to the information age, their patients may be very educated about their health, and they don't feel defensive when confronted with a knowledgeable patient in their office. They'll be intrigued by what you have to report and are interested in your ideas. If you feel belittled by your health-care professional, it might be time to switch, finding someone more willing to work with you and respect the self-advocacy work you're doing.

What if you need medications? By all means, take them when they are necessary. They can be lifesaving. It's a silly myth that doctors are all in the pocket of the pharmaceutical industry and just want to "push pills." Most are practicing medicine the very best way they know how. At the same time, be sure that you and your doctor both know the potential side effects of any medication you are taking, including nutrient depletions and potential drug-supplement interactions. In Appendix, 4 "Drug-Nutrient Depletions and Interactions," I'll cover some of the more common pharmaceutical drugs and how they interact with key nutrients and nutritional supplements.

Ideally, I would like to see more teamwork between doctors and other health professionals. I believe that pharmacists should deepen their training in dietary supplements, as they are a logical choice for counseling patients about possible adverse interactions between supplements and drugs. I definitely believe there should be greater referral and collaboration with dietitians and nutritionists to help patients figure out what type of nutritional program is best for them based upon their age, gender, medical history, and personal preferences. Nutrition and lifestyle medicine should be offered to and by health-care professionals across all specialties—chiropractors, nurse practitioners, acupuncturists, naturopaths, psychologists, and so on—as they are fundamental to improving the health of our nation. I'm glad that more and more, doctors are getting additional training in "integrative medicine" and learning when and how to refer to an acupuncturist, massage therapist, or dietitian; how to do motivational interviewing, and so on. I believe integrative medicine training leads to happier patients *and* health-care providers. And I also think it is a good idea to have a range of practitioners to work with, depending upon your own personal health situation.

RX FROM DR. LOW DOG

R℞ How to Find a Physician Trained in Integrative Medicine

Check to see whether your physician is board certified in Integrative Medicine through the American Association of Physician *(www .aapsus.org)*.

Check the following training programs to see whether there is a practitioner trained in Integrative Medicine near you:

Academy of Integrative Health & Medicine *(www.aihm.org)*
Arizona Center for Integrative Medicine *(www.integrativemedicine .arizona.edu)*

To find a dietitian trained in integrative dietetics, visit: *http:// integrativerd.org/resources/find-an-integrative-rd/*

OWN YOUR HEALTH

Taking charge of your health means knowing about the most important nutrients you need, and about the ones that are most likely to be able to help you achieve the state of physical wellness you desire. My goal in writing this book has been to help empower you with knowledge about vitamins, minerals, and specific nutraceuticals that could help you in your quest to remain energetic, fit, and feeling great.

Your Food Journal

Keeping a food journal can be an excellent strategy for evaluating the nutritional status of your daily dietary intake. It can also help you gain some interesting insights into what drives your eating habits and whether there are certain foods that don't quite sit right with you. All it requires is for you to write down all the foods and beverages you consume, and the portion sizes, for two to three days. Make sure you include added salt, ketchup, mustard, and other condiments. Note the times that you ate and whether you were eating a meal or a snack. In the notes section, record how you felt before and after eating. Did you feel gassy or bloated? Did your mood change? Did you feel tired and fatigued before or after eating? Do you get a headache when you don't eat or when you eat or drink certain foods or beverages?

By creating a food journal, you will have an easier time calculating your nutrient intake, which will help you to determine which nutritional supplements would be best for you and if so, how much. Keep your food journal for at least two days. If you are working with a nutritionist, doctor, or other health-care providers, show them your journal. You can also use on-line trackers to calculate your nutritional intake. My favorite is My Fitness Pal (*www.myfitnesspal.com*).

Here are some examples of serving sizes:

- 3 ounces of meat is about the size of a deck of cards.
- 1 ounce of cheese is about size of four dice.
- 1 cup of vegetables, 1 cup of dry cereal, and 1 cup of yogurt are each equal to the size of a baseball.
- One slice of bread is a serving size, one serving of pancakes is one pancake the size of a CD or DVD.
- One serving of whole fruit or pasta is about the size of a tennis ball.
- 1 teaspoon is the length from the tip of the thumb to the first joint.
- 1 tablespoon of salad dressing is about the size of a silver dollar.

Time	Meal or Snack?	What You Ate	Notes/How You Felt

Appendix 2

Your Personalized Supplements Chart

O kay, so now you've learned how supplements might be beneficial for maintaining and supporting your health and wellness goals; the next step is to figure out which ones might be right for you. To create your own personalized supplement plan, spend some time working your way through the following exercise

First, write down all your current medications, over-the-counter medications, and supplements and when you take them. Next, go to Appendix 4, "Drug-Nutrient Interactions," to see whether you need to be aware of any interactions or timing issues. For some drugs, it is very important to take them at least two hours apart from certain nutrients, particularly minerals. Many medications can deplete your body of important nutrients, so check to see whether your medication is one of them. If so, make a notation in your list.

Next, use the table on page XXX to see whether you should be considering supplementing with—or adjusting your current level or form of—any other vitamins, minerals or nutraceuticals based upon your lifestyle, age, or specific health concern. Make a note of those in your list.

Using this information, you can now begin to put together your own personal plan. You probably want to include a multivitamin-mineral supplement. Do you need iron, or should you purchase a multivitamin-mineral supplement that omits it? What forms of key nutrients are you looking for and how much: methylcobalamin for vitamin B12? pyridoxal 5'-phosphate for vitamin B6? Are you eating fish? If not, maybe you want to add some marine omega-3 fatty acids. How much EPA and DHA should you be looking for? What about vitamin D? Unless you're a strict vegan, look for vitamin D3, usually listed as cholecalciferol on the label. In the first column of the chart on page XX, first make a list of the medications and supplements that are most important for you. In the second column, include important information about the form and serving size, or dosage, for your specific

Supplement name	Dosage (unit and amt. per unit)	Early a.m.	Breakfast	

situation—for example, 1 tablet, 2 capsules, and so on, plus the amount per unit, so you are really aware of how much of each medication or supplement you take per dosage.

Now, in the remaining columns, lay out a typical day, distributing the medications and supplements across the times of day you will be using them. What time would take your medication and what time you would take your supplements? Here are some suggestions: You'll usually want to take your multivitamin-mineral supplement with breakfast, fish oil or omega-3 and vitamin D with dinner or another fatty meal, your melatonin 1 to 2 hours before bedtime, and magnesium when you slide into the sheets. Put a check mark in each box for when you take a medication or a supplement. The pattern resulting represents your daily supplements plan. Look carefully at your original list and double-check all of your notes. Go back and read the specific sections that have to do with the nutrients you are most interested in. And of course, if you have any concerns or questions, talk to your pharmacist or health-care practitioner.

	2 hrs. after breakfast	Lunch	2 hrs. after lunch	Dinner	Bedtime

Appendix 3

Laboratory Tests

I wish I could say that your health-care provider is routinely ensuring that you are not deficient in key nutrients but that just isn't the case. The idea of nutrient testing is just not on the mind of most health-care professionals, in no small part because of the persistent messages telling us that we're getting everything we need in our diet. By now, after reading this book, I hope you realize that probably isn't true. As a physician, I follow recommended guidelines for laboratory testing for cholesterol, blood sugar, hepatitis C, and HIV and screening for cervical, breast, colorectal, and skin cancers, as well as osteoporosis. I also recommend regular vision and hearing tests and make sure my patients are keeping their immunizations up to date. Screening guidelines are for the general population and are based on population data. However, I don't take care of populations; I take care of individuals. I must use my clinical judgment when it comes to checking thyroid, ordering advanced heart testing, screening for anemia, and so on. And I believe that this should also include being alert for possible nutrient deficiencies and ordering laboratory tests when appropriate.

Let's say you have had diabetes for nine years and have been taking metformin for five of those years. I believe it is totally reasonable to order an HgA1C test to see how stable your blood sugar has been over the course of the past 60 to 90 days, and also consider checking your levels of vitamin B12 and magnesium, and possibly thiamine and vitamin B6. Diabetes can deplete the body of these critical nutrients and long-term use of metformin can lead to B12 deficiency. Monitoring your blood sugar stability is *very* important but it is only the tip of the iceberg. It's the iceberg that's under the water that you can't easily see that is often the most dangerous.

As I mentioned earlier, I check blood levels for a range of things: cholesterol, blood sugar, potassium, etc. That's because I have no way of knowing what your cholesterol is simply by looking at you. It's the same thing when it comes to vitamin D. Some of my patients who've been taking 1,000 IU per day of vitamin D3 for years were found to have really low serum vitamin D levels when they were checked. Many walk around without symptoms, but others complain of pain in their lower back, hips and/or thighs, all of which can be signs of osteomalacia, a condition in which your bone-building process is impaired, weakening bones, causing them to ache, increasing the likelihood of fracture, and making muscles feel weak. According to data from the CDC, 23 million Americans have blood levels of vitamin D that indicate *severe* deficiency that could cause rickets in a child or osteomalacia in an adult. I recommend 2,000 IU per day for most teens and adults, but as I always say, the amount you really need to take is the amount that will get your blood to the level recommended by the Endocrine Society, at or above 30 ng/mL. And only a blood test will tell you that.

Metformin, as I mentioned previously, is only one example of the many medications that can deplete important nutrients. I agree it should be the responsibility of the prescriber to make sure he or she is keeping a watchful eye on your diet and monitoring for any signs/symptoms that might suggest a nutrient deficiency. But prescribers just aren't trained in thinking about the consequences of drug-induced nutrient depletion. Unfortunately, for now, you have to be your own advocate. Please review Appendix 4, "Drug-Nutrient Depletion and Interaction," to determine whether you might be at risk for any particular nutrient deficiency. If so, talk to your health-care provider about testing or consider ordering the test yourself.

When I went through medical school, we studied genetics and learned about the most common and dangerous genetic disorders. But at that time, we had no way of knowing that there were such vast differences in the genetic makeup of the American population. Differences that influence how nutrients are absorbed, activated, and metabolized. This is just one more example of how one size does not fit all, especially when it comes to our nutritional needs. At this time, it's not common practice to do genetic testing for the metabolism of drugs or nutrients, though there will probably come a day when this will be standard practice. But without this testing there isn't any way of knowing whether you are one of the 20 to 50 percent of people who have a genetic variation that affects the metabolism of certain nutrients. The only way to know if you have enough of a specific nutrient is through laboratory testing.

I'm sure some health-care providers will frown upon me including this section. After all, many of you reading this section are not health-care professionals. What will you do with this information? Well, if you do order some of your own laboratory tests, I want you to take the results with you to your next health-care appointment and discuss them. If they are in the normal range, that's great! However, if some of your lab tests come back abnormal, you will need to work with your provider to find out why you are deficient and create a plan for getting them back in the normal range. I believe that information is powerful and that an informed patient is an empowered patient.

You do *not* need to check all the nutrients that follow. Just focus on your particular situation. If you are a vegan, over 60 years old, have a specific medical condition, take certain medications, or have certain dietary restrictions; you might want to consider checking those specific nutrients for which you might be at greatest risk for deficiency. I have migraines and take 600 mg of magnesium every night. Imagine how surprised I was that my red blood cell magnesium came back on the low end of normal even at this dose! I had it checked because I've been taking this dose for years and was afraid I might be getting *too much*. There just isn't any way to really know what your levels are without checking them.

It's important to recognize that laboratories around the country can use different units of measurements. I have tried to include those used by the Centers for Disease Control, as well as those most commonly used in the U.S. If the test says that it is done in the fasting state, that means overnight fasting of 12 to 14 hours. All of the reference ranges I have provided below are for adults (aged 18 and older) and do not reflect ranges for children or teens.

Vitamin A: The normal range for serum vitamin A is 32.5 to 78.0 mcg/dL. When the serum concentration is less than 20 mcg/dL (<0.7 mmol/L), it reflects a very significant vitamin A deficiency. Because vitamin A can also be toxic, you don't want to go over the top end of the range. An ideal range is probably 45 to 65 mcg/dL. This test is done in the fasting state.

Vitamin B1 (thiamine): Whole blood or red blood cell testing of thiamine diphosphate is considered to be the most accurate

R℞ FROM DR. LOW DOG

Ordering Your Own Lab Tests

To check your blood levels of nutrients, such as vitamins B12 or D, iron, or magnesium, you don't necessarily need to have your health-care provider order them. A major U.S. drugstore chain is experimenting with offering their customers the opportunity to order basic lab tests quickly and at a lower cost; often, results are received within just a few hours. As more people begin taking charge of their own health, I suspect we'll see more clever innovations like this one.

I also believe private lab testing will become more popular in the future as patients face increasingly higher deductibles with their health insurance plans. If it costs $300 through your health-care provider to get the same labs done that can be purchased independently for $152 and you are paying for it—it's kind of a no-brainer. If your physician won't order your test, or your health insurance won't cover the tests, or if you have a high deductible and are looking to save money, you can use online labs, such as My Medlab (*www.mymedlab.com*), Health Check USA (*www.health-checkusa.com*) or WellnessFX (*www.wellnessfx.com*), to order your own home-based tests. You just go into one of the test centers listed on the website to have the labs drawn, which are then sent to a nationally accredited laboratory. Your results are available on line generally within 24 to 72 hours.

way to measure thiamine. Plasma or serum thiamine tests do not accurately reflect the state of thiamine in the body. The normal range is 90 to 180 nmol/L, 70 to 90 nmol/L is considered marginal deficiency, and anything below 70 nmol/L indicates deficiency. This test is done in the fasting state.

Vitamin B2 (riboflavin): Riboflavin status is best assessed using a test called the erythrocyte glutathione reductase activity coefficient (EGRAC). If the level is greater than 1.4, it indicates deficiency. A level of 1.2 to 1.4 indicates marginal status, and less than 1.2 means you have sufficient levels. Some labs do not offer this test and use a fasting serum test to check riboflavin. Serum riboflavin has a very wide range for what is considered normal: 1 to 19 mcg/L. If using this laboratory measure, an ideal range is probably closer to 10 to 19 mcg/L.

Vitamin B3 (niacin): The normal range for serum niacin is 0.5 to 8.45 mcg/mL. This is a very large reference range, an ideal range would be somewhere in the midpoint: 4 to 7 mcg/mL.

Vitamin B5 (pantothenic acid): Tests for pantothenic acid levels in blood or urine are available but are very seldom ordered, as deficiency is extremely rare. The normal range for this test is 37 to 147 µg/L. Do not take any supplemental pantothenic acid within 24 hours of the test.

Vitamin B6 (pyridoxine): Serum pyridoxal 5'-phosphate (PLP) is considered the very best indicator of B6 status. Less than 20 nmol/L is deficient; a level between 20 to 30 nmol/L indicates marginal status. You want your level to be greater than 30 nmol/L. Do not take any supplemental pyridoxine within 24 hours of the test. This test is done in the fasting state.

Biotin (B7): A serum biotin can be ordered, though the "normal" reference range is extremely wide: 221 to 3,004 pg/mL. Obviously, a midpoint is probably indicative of sufficiency. Another test that is sometimes used is to check the urine for biotin excretion, as low urinary excretion indicates low body stores.

Vitamin B9 (folate): There are two primary ways to evaluate folate levels in the body. Serum folate reflects recent intake of folate; blood must be drawn when you are fasting. Red blood cell folate is a better indicator of long-term folate storage, though the test itself may not be as analytically accurate as the serum level. The CDC says a *serum* folate level less than 3 ng/mL indicates a deficiency, as does a *red blood cell* folate level less than 95 ng/mL. However, some experts believe a more accurate cutoff for red blood cell folate deficiency should be anything less than 140 ng/mL. You can also get too much folate, especially from eating lots of fortified foods and taking supplements. While the range is 3.0 to 17 ng/mL, a midrange level is probably optimal: 9 to 13 ng/mL.

Note: Homocysteine and methylmalonic acid (MMA) are usually ordered when assessing megaloblastic anemia (the anemia caused by folate or B12 deficiency). In folate deficiency, homocysteine levels are elevated, while MMA levels are normal.

The normal level for homocysteine is less than 14 to 16 (different cutoffs are used), but ideally you'd like your level to be between 6 and 9.

Vitamin B12 (cobalamin): While a serum B12 level less than 200 pg/mL is considered the cutoff point for deficiency, subclinical deficiency is seen when B12 levels are in the 200 to 400 pg/mL (ng/L) range. A more specific test for B12 deficiency is the serum MMA test. Elevated MMA occurs early in vitamin B12 deficiency, and is a better indicator of B12 status. Using the MMA cutoff of greater than 271 nmol/L, the CDC found that more than 18 million Americans are deficient in vitamin B12.

Note: When B12 levels are low and MMA is elevated, an intrinsic factor blocking antibody (IFBA) test is often ordered to determine if the cells in your stomach are making intrinsic factor, which is needed to bind B12 for absorption in the small intestine.

Vitamin C: Serum or plasma ascorbic acid levels less than 11.4 µmol/L indicate deficiency. Levels between 11.4 and 50 µmol/L indicate suboptimal status. Other reference ranges: normal 0.6 to 2.0 mg/dl, with anything less than 0.6 mg/dl indicating suboptimal or deficient status. The test is done in the fasting state.

Vitamin D: The optimal time for vitamin D testing is during the winter. The most accurate vitamin D test is the 25(OH)D test. The Centers for Disease Control used a cutoff of 20 ng/mL (50 nmol/L) for insufficiency. However, in the Endocrine Society Clinical Guidelines, the goal is to achieve a vitamin D level equal to or greater than 30 ng/mL (75 nmol/L). If deficient/insufficient, the current recommendations are to take 50,000 IU of vitamin D3 *one time per week* for eight weeks and then have your level rechecked. Do *not* just continue to take 50,000 IU per week! For most of us, a range of 30 to 50 ng/mL (75–125 nmol/L) is optimal and once levels are corrected, taking 1,500 to 2,000 IU per day of vitamin D3 should be adequate.

Note: Can your vitamin D level be too high? We don't know. But some experts believe a 25(OH)D level equal to or greater than 80 ng/mL (200 nmol/L) could be dangerous. My recommendation is to stay within the 30 to 50 ng/mL range.

Vitamin E: Serum vitamin E levels less than 500 micrograms/ dL indicates deficiency. Other reference range: A level less than 4 mg/L indicates the need for supplementation, whereas a level greater than 40 mg/L indicates excess intake. Discontinue vitamin

E supplementation at least 24 hours before the test. This test is done in the fasting state.

Vitamin K: Levels of vitamin K1 can be assessed with a fasting blood specimen. The normal reference range for adults is 0.1 to 2.2 ng/mL. However, with levels below 0.5 ng/mL, one can see impaired blood clotting. Discontinue vitamin K supplements at least 24 hours before the test.

Calcium: Calcium levels can be checked with a simple blood test. Normal range for adults is 8.9 to 10.1 mg/dL. Any level that is over or under this range should be further evaluated by a qualified health-care professional.

Coenzyme Q10: Low levels of CoQ10 have been associated with numerous neurological diseases, as well as diabetes and heart disease. Normal values for those over the age of 18 are 433 to 1,532 mcg/L. Aim for a level around 1,000 mcg/L.

Iodine: A spot urine iodine test is an easy way to test for iodine deficiency, which is defined as a median urine iodine (UI) concentration of 100 to 199 mcg/L for the general population. The World Health Organization recommends that the median UI in pregnancy should be 150 to 249 mcg/L. A level greater than 300 mcg/L is excessive and could increase your risk for autoimmune thyroid disease.

Iron: Ferritin is considered to be one of the best indicators for iron deficiency. Anyone who has low serum ferritin and low serum iron has iron deficiency.

In men ferritin levels less than 24 mcg/L, and in women less than 11 mcg/L, usually indicate iron deficiency. Iron levels in men less than 50 mcg/dL, and in women less than 35 mcg/dL, indicate iron deficiency. (Normal range for iron in men is 50–150 mcg/dL and women 35–145 mcg/dL.) Iron can be toxic in excess. Higher than normal levels may indicate hemochromatosis, a genetic disorder that causes the body to store excess iron. When iron is low or high, it should prompt a further evaluation with a qualified health-care professional.

Magnesium: Serum tests for magnesium are what are commonly used to screen for magnesium. They can tell you how much magnesium is in your blood but not what is in your cells. Your serum level can be in the normal range while your cells are starving. The most accurate test for assessing intracellular magnesium status is the erythrocyte or red blood cell magnesium test. The normal reference range at my local lab is 3.5 to 7.1 mg/dL; your lab may have different values. Lower levels indicate deficiency. The test is done in the fasting state.

Omega-3 fatty acids: It is possible to test your omega-3 levels so that you know if you are in the right range with diet and/or supplements. The omega-3 index is a measurement of EPA and DHA as a percent of total fatty acids in your red blood cell membranes. While there is debate regarding the optimal level, an omega-3 index greater than 6 percent is desirable, with some experts believing 8 percent or higher is optimal.

Potassium: Health-care providers often monitor potassium because medications can deplete this vital nutrient. The normal range is 3.6 to 5.2 mmol/L. Potassium levels less than 3 mmol/L are accompanied by neuromuscular symptoms, indicating a significant deficiency; a level less than 2.5 mmol/L is potentially life-threatening. Too much potassium is also very dangerous. A level greater than 6 mmol/L is considered life-threatening.

Selenium: Selenium status can be evaluated by plasma selenium or erythrocyte selenium concentration. Plasma levels of 70 to 150 ng/mL are considered to be within the normal range. When levels fall below 40 ng/mL, glutathione (a vitally important antioxidant in the body) is no longer active. Selenium can also be toxic. An ideal range is somewhere between 90 and 130 ng/mL.

Zinc: While serum zinc levels are used in an attempt to assess status, the test is not considered very accurate or reliable. However, given that, normal serum zinc levels are considered to be in the range of 0.66 to 1.10 mcg/mL. Some people believe the zinc test taste is an effective way to assess zinc levels: If you can taste liquid zinc, it's said that you are not zinc deficient. However, but there is very little evidence that this is a reliable test for deficiency in zinc.

Drug–Nutrient Depletions and Interactions

There's no way around it: America is a pill-popping nation. More than half of Americans take at least one prescription per day and 20 percent take three or more. That number will only grow as more and more of us are battling diabetes, cancer, and heart, respiratory, and autoimmune diseases. While many of these drugs are lifesaving, I believe that we rely too heavily on them, and we seldom talk about the critical nutrients that can be lost as a consequence of their use. Throughout this book, I have tried to show just how intertwined and interconnected vitamins and minerals are in the beautiful biochemical dance that is life. It's almost impossible for you to become depleted in one nutrient without that deficiency affecting other nutrients and bodily processes. Yet, very few health-care professionals are routinely checking nutrient levels and even fewer discuss the potential for deficiencies with their patients, with the exception of potassium and diuretic use. This is why I have created this appendix: so you can be knowledgeable about what impact the drugs you are taking might be having on your nutritional status.

BATTLING DISEASES, DEPRESSION, AND DEFICIENCIES: Glenn's Story of Improved Health

Glenn was in his 70s when I first met him. He had been struggling with cancer for many years, and when I saw him for his initial visit, he was tired, depressed, and experiencing significant tingling and numbness in his feet and calves. He told me he had lost about 4 inches in height and gained 25 pounds, and that his lower back and hips hurt, he felt weak when he walked, he'd lost a tooth, his gums bled when he brushed them, he bruised easily, he felt that his mind was in a fog, and he tossed and turned for hours before falling asleep because of restless legs and cramping in his calves, which only compounded his fatigue and inability to think clearly. He told me several times that he realized he was getting old and that he knew it was "probably normal to feel this way". When I asked if he had a pastor or counselor he could talk to about his feelings, he told me that he "didn't know anyone." His doctor had given him a prescription for Zoloft for depression but he said he never took it. After listening to Glenn's story, carefully reviewing his medical chart and labs, and doing a physical exam, I believed there were a number of things that could be done to improve his quality of life.

For more than 13 years, Glenn had been on medications to block the testosterone that was fueling his prostate cancer. During that time, no one had ever checked his bone density or his vitamin D levels, in spite of the fact that virtually all men on this type of therapy will develop osteoporosis after this length of time. When he had developed heartburn during his chemotherapy six years previously, he was placed on 40 mg of Nexium, a drug for lowering stomach acid and reflux that he was still taking, though he admitted he lived with horrible gas, bloating, and frequent diarrhea. He'd been given a small dose of prednisone as part of his treatment, which caused weight gain and his blood sugar to rise. He had then been placed on 850 mg twice daily of the diabetes drug metformin. Even though Glenn appeared depressed, and this was clearly noted in his chart, no one had ever referred him for counseling.

After doing some detective work and getting a DEXA scan to determine the state of his bone health, we uncovered a whole range of problems. His B6, B12, iron, magnesium, and vitamin C levels came back extremely low. Tests showed his vitamin D level was 8 ng/mL, which indicated osteomalacia. Osteomalacia impairs the bone building process and causes weakening of the bones, increasing his risk for fracture but also causing bone pain, especially in the lower back, pelvis, and hips, as well as muscle weakness. Glenn complained of back and hip pain and muscle weakness. His DEXA scan showed significant osteoporosis. His hs-CRP, a test that indicates how much inflammation is in the body, came back quite elevated.

Unfortunately, Glenn's case is more common than anyone would like to admit. While his cancer had been kept "in check," his quality of life had plummeted, in part because of the nutritional deficiencies related to his disease and the medications he was taking. The combination of Nexium and metformin had caused him to become severely deficient in B12 over time. His diet, diabetes, and cancer drove the inflammation in his body, which caused his B6 levels to fall. Vitamins B6 and B12 are critically important for the production of neurotransmitters in the brain that are responsible for mood and pleasure. Low levels increase the risk for depression and impair cognition, attention, and memory. These vitamins also help in the production of myelin, the protective covering of our nerves, which explains why a deficiency can lead to tingling and burning in our extremities. His low levels of vitamins B6 and D, which are necessary for the production of melatonin, may have contributed to his poor sleep.

Nexium reduced his ability to other key nutrients, as well. Without sufficient stomach acid, Glenn was unable to absorb the non-heme iron in his diet, and vitamin C was being destroyed by the high stomach pH. His magnesium levels plummeted. His B12 deficiency and low iron levels led to anemia, leaving him tired and fatigued. Should his doctors have predicted that this might happen as a result of his medications? The FDA notified prescribers in 2011 that proton pump inhibitors, such as Nexium, could cause serious magnesium deficiency. Low magnesium reduces our ability to manage our blood sugar, aggravating diabetes. It also causes muscle cramping, which Glenn was experiencing. It increases inflammation and contributes to osteoporosis. His low vitamin C was contributing to his bleeding gums, easy bruising and fatigue. His iron deficiency most certainly was contributing to his restless legs.

When stomach acid is inhibited, over time the bacteria in the large intestine migrate up into the small intestine, where they disrupt the microbiome; consume vitamin B12; and cause gas, bloating, and diarrhea. Diarrhea further reduces absorption of fat-soluble vitamins A, D, and E. This condition is referred to as small intestinal bacterial overgrowth (SIBO). I referred him to a gastroenterologist who diagnosed Glenn with SIBO and treated him with an antibiotic, which stopped the diarrhea. To restore balance to his gut microflora, he started taking a high-quality probiotic containing *Lactobacillus* and *Bifidobacterium*.

I wish I could say that everything got better overnight but it didn't. Even with his taking 50,000 IU per week of vitamin D3, more than four months passed before his vitamin D level rose to 30 ng/mL. Glenn's vitamin D level was so low that he could not absorb the calcium needed for strong bones, healthy muscle contractions, and nerve conduction. As you'll recall, vitamin D is critical for preventing osteoporosis, as well as for heart and immune health. When levels fall, people experience muscle weakness and pain. Why had no one ever thought to check his vitamin D level?

It took almost three months to wean Glenn off his Nexium, using 5 mg of melatonin every night to treat his reflux. With continued use of melatonin, and after correcting his SIBO, he did not experience a return of his heartburn. Because of his depression and age, I gave him weekly B12 injections for one month, along with a high-potency B-complex supplement that provided 100 mg of the active form of vitamin B6 and 500 mcg of vitamin B12, as well as a food-based iron supplement with vitamin C, and 400 mg of magnesium. Glenn began to feel an improvement with his energy, memory, and mood. Unfortunately, Glenn's neuropathy, or nerve damage, in his feet and lower legs, which was related to the diabetes and the nutritional deficiencies, was long-standing and could not be reversed but was improved with prescription medication.

All the time we were taking care of his nutrients, we were also addressing his diet. Glenn began eating more protein and followed a Mediterranean diet that featured low-glycemic foods (foods that do not cause a rapid rise in sugar). He replaced afternoon soda pop with a variety of naturally flavored green teas. He lost 15 pounds and was able to decrease his dose of metformin by half within six months. He was able to tolerate short repetitions of arm weights that helped counter some of his muscle loss. I referred him to a psychologist in town who works with people living with cancer. They hit it off very well and Glenn shared many of the feelings he'd been living with for more than 20 years as he dealt with his cancer, depression, limited finances, and deep concerns about how his wife of 50 years would survive without him.

TRUSTING HER INSTINCTS INSTEAD OF "NORMAL" LAB REPORTS:
Pat's Story of Improved Health

You may think Glenn's is an extreme or unusual case. I'm sorry to say that it is not. Pat was a 57-year-old woman who came to my office with symptoms of fatigue, muscle cramps, and an altered sense of taste and smell. Her blood pressure was creeping up even though she was taking her blood pressure medication, and she'd recently been told she was prediabetic, that is, insulin resistant and on the path toward developing full-blown type 2 diabetes. She was concerned because she hadn't changed her diet, she watched her salt intake, and couldn't understand why she wasn't feeling well. She wanted an integrative medicine provider to evaluate her after her primary care provider told her all her tests were normal and that she was fine. She didn't *feel* fine.

The thiazide diuretic Pat had been taking for her blood pressure for the last couple of years was a good choice, as she'd had some loss of bone density after going through menopause and thiazides help the body retain calcium. Her gynecologist had put her on 600 mg of calcium twice a day along with 1,000 IU of vitamin D3. Because thiazides can cause a loss of sodium and potassium, her primary care physician had closely monitored and corrected these when necessary. However, thiazides also deplete the body of magnesium, zinc, B-vitamins, and other key nutrients. I noted that her serum magnesium test performed six months earlier showed her magnesium level was at the low end of the normal range. There is no quick and easy lab test for zinc, but zinc deficiency causes fatigue, an altered sense of taste and smell, and poor wound healing.

After I got more information, some of what Pat was experiencing started to make sense. Her vitamin D level came back at 21 ng/mL, lower than the 30 ng/mL needed to maintain healthy bones and overall health. She was surprised to find that her vitamin D level was not "normal," as her doctor had told her. I explained that physicians disagree about what the optimal level should be and that I followed the Endocrine Society's guidelines of achieving a level of greater than 30 ng/mL, especially because she had some loss in bone density and a family history of osteoporosis. This is why you want to know what *your* vitamin D level is! It's also why you can't assume that taking 1,000 IU per day of vitamin D will normalize your levels. She took 50,000 IU of vitamin D3 once a week for eight weeks and then we rechecked her level, which was 32 ng/mL. She continued on a maintenance dose of 2,000 IU per day.

We calculated her dietary calcium to be roughly 1,300 mg per day. Pat was somewhat skeptical when I told her that she was getting enough calcium in her diet and asked her to discontinue her supplements. She looked at me and said sternly, "The National Osteoporosis Association says women over 50 should be taking

1,200 mg per day of calcium." I reassured her that she was correct and that she needed 1,200 mg calcium from *all* sources and that she should only supplement what she wasn't getting in her diet. She was currently getting around 2,500 mg per day, 500 mg more per day than the upper limit for her age. I then explained that she also needed vitamins D, K, magnesium and a number of trace minerals to maintain healthy bones. Calcium is just one part of a complex puzzle. We found a multiple vitamin-mineral supplement that provided 150 mcg of vitamin K, 25 mg of zinc and no iron (important because women should not take iron supplements after their menstrual periods have stopped).

We discovered Pat's red blood cell magnesium levels were quite low. This was most likely because (1) her dietary intake of magnesium was low (about 280 mg per day), (2) she was taking high doses of calcium that block the absorption of magnesium (and other trace minerals), and (3) she was on a thiazide diuretic that causes magnesium to be lost in the urine. Low magnesium increases the risk for insulin resistance (remember, she had recently been diagnosed as prediabetic). It also increases the risk for postmenopausal osteoporosis (she has osteopenia already), elevation in blood pressure (her blood pressure had been creeping up even on the medication), muscle cramps, and more. She started taking 400 mg of magnesium citrate at night before bedtime.

We also worked on her diet and got her started on an exercise program that she would stick with. Pat was a motivated woman and because of all of her hard work, she kept her blood pressure under control, avoided diabetes, and maintained her bone health. Even her taste returned to normal. Listening to her instincts, and to her body's signals that something wasn't right, instead of simply trusting her physician's interpretation of seemingly normal lab reports, paid off for Pat.

I could go on with more cases, but I think you are starting to get the point. Medications have multiple benefits and multiple downsides, including depleting your body of key nutrients it requires to function. Clearly, not everyone is going to have the same risk for a nutrient depletion given differences in diet, lifestyle, and genetics. But the longer you take a drug, and the more drugs you take, the greater your risk will be. It is often through optimizing essential nutrients—which you've learned about in this book—that your health improves. Taking St. John's wort for depression is no better than taking Zoloft if the problem is B6 or B12 deficiency. Taking ginseng or rhodiola for energy won't help if you don't have enough iron. Focus on the foundation of nutrition, know your body, and partner with health-care professionals rather than look to them for every answer and I think you'll be far better off than if you simply assumed that all health-care providers know about your personal nutritional needs.

And finally, as your health conditions change and symptoms cease, don't simply stop taking the medications you are using. Talk to your health-care provider before making that decision.

Common Prescription Drugs and Nutritional Interactions

In the first column of this table, the generic name of each drug is followed in parentheses by brand-name versions of the drug.

Drug	Nutrients Depleted	
Analgesics and Anti-inflammatories		
Acetaminophen (Tylenol)		
Aspirin	Vitamins B1 (thiamine), B7 (biotin), B9 (folate) and C; iron, zinc	
Nonsteroidal Anti-inflammatory Drugs		
Diclofenac (Cataflam, Voltaren) Diflunisal (Dolobid) Etodolac (Lodine) Ibuprofen (Advil, Midol IB, Motrin, Nuprin) Indomethacin (Indocin) Meclofenamate (Meclomen) Nabumetone (Relafen) Naproxen (Aleve, Naprosyn) Oxaprozin (Daypro) Piroxicam (Feldene) Sulindac (Clinoril)	Vitamins B9 (folate) and C; iron, melatonin, zinc	
Other		
Pentazocine (Talwin) Meperidine (Demerol) Tramadol (Ultram)		
Anticoagulants		
Warfarin (Coumadin)	CoQ10, calcium, magnesium, potassium, zinc, vitamin B9 (folate)	
Anticonvulsant (Antiseizure) Drugs		
Carbamazepine (Atelol, Epitol, Tegretol)	Vitamins B7 (biotin), B9 (folate), D, E and K; calcium	
Phenobarbital (Luminal, Solfoton) Primidone (Mysoline)	Vitamins B5 (pantothenic acid), B7 (biotin), B9 (folate), B12 (cobalamin), D, E and K; calcium (possibly l-carnitine)	
Phenytoin (Dilantin) Fosphenytoin (Cerebyx)	Vitamins B1 (thiamine), B2 (riboflavin), B3 (niacin), B5 (pantothenic acid), B7 (biotin), B9 (folate), B12 (cobalamin), D, E and K; calcium, zinc (possibly l-carnitine)	
Valproic acid and derivatives (Depacon, Depakene, Depakote)	Vitamins B3 (niacin), B9 (folate), calcium, zinc, selenium, (possibly l-carnitine)	
Anti-infectives		
Antibiotics	All antibiotics deplete beneficial bacteria and vitamin K.	

Interactions	Notes
	In general, take these drugs with food to reduce gastric irritation. Alcohol can further aggravate gut.
Vitamin C reduces urinary excretion of acetaminophen, increasing risk for toxicity. Do not take >500 mg of vitamin C per day. Taking aspirin before taking high-dose vitamin B3 (niacin) can reduce flushing.	If taking regularly, be cautious with alcohol as they can both damage the liver. Can deplete glutathione; ensure adequate intake of B-vitamins and SAMe. Increases urinary secretion of vitamin C. Damage to the GI mucosa can lead to iron deficiency due to chronic blood loss. Consider taking 200 mg of vitamin C twice daily.
Omega-3 fatty acids may protect the stomach.	These drugs inhibit some folate dependent enzymes. Damage to the GI mucosa can lead to iron deficiency due to chronic blood loss. Consider taking 200–400 mcg per day of methylfolate, 200 mg of vitamin C twice daily, omega-3 fatty acids daily, and 1–3 mg per day of melatonin if having poor sleep.
Don't take these medications with SAMe or 5-HTP; serotonin syndrome could result.	
Take drug 2 hours before or 4 hours after taking magnesium, iron, vitamin B3 (niacin), and/or zinc. Do not exceed 200 IU of vitamin E.	A multivitamin with no more than the DV of vitamin K is generally acceptable if taken every day at the same time and blood tests for coagulation remain in the normal range. Always talk to your health-care provider before taking a new supplement, as *many* can interact with warfarin.
Take drug 2 hours before or 4 hours after calcium supplements.	Decreased absorption and/or increased metabolism of folate, biotin, and vitamins D and K. Levels should be closely monitored. Multivitamin-mineral strongly encouraged.
Take drug 2 hours before or 4 hours after calcium supplements.	Decreased absorption and/or increased metabolism of folate, biotin, and vitamins D and K. Levels should be closely monitored. Multivitamin-mineral strongly encouraged. May increase the need for vitamin C; consider taking 200 mg twice daily.
Don't exceed the DV of vitamin B6 without talking to health-care provider. Higher doses may reduce effectiveness of drug.	Decreased absorption and/or increased metabolism of folate, biotin and vitamins D and K. Levels should be closely monitored. Multivitamin-mineral strongly encouraged. May cause carnitine deficiency. Consider 1,000 mg per day of acetyl-l-carnitine.
Take probiotics during and at least 3–4 months after antibiotic therapy. If taking antibiotics for more than 10 days, supplement with the DV of vitamin K.	Taking antibiotics on an empty stomach enhances absorption; taking with food reduces stomach upset.

Drug	Nutrients Depleted	
Cephalosporins		
Cefprozil (Cefzil) Cefuroxime (Ceftin) Loracarbef (Lorabid)	Vitamins B2 (riboflavin), B7 (biotin), B9 (folate), B12 (cobalamin)	
Macrolides		
Azithromycin (Zithromax) Clarithromycin (Biaxin) Erythromycin (E-mycin)	Vitamins B2 (riboflavin), B7 (biotin), B9 (folate), B12 (cobalamin)	
Quinolones		
Ciprofloxacin (Cipro) Lomefloxacin (Maxaquin) Levofloxacin (Levaquin) Norfloxacin (Noroxin) Ofloxacin (Floxin) Sparfloxacin (Zagam) Trovafloxacin (Trovan)	Vitamins B2 (riboflavin), B9 (folate), B12 (cobalamin); biotin, iron, calcium.	
Penicillins		
Carbenicillin (Geocillin) Mezlocillin (Mezlin) Penicillin G sodium (Pfizerpen) Ticarcillin (Ticar)	Vitamin B6 (pyridoxine) and potassium	
Tetracyclines		

Doxycycline (Doryx, Doxy caps,
    Doxychel, Monodox, Periostat)
Minocycline (Dynacin, Vectrin)
Oxytetracycline (Terramycin,
    Uri-Tet)
Tetracycline (Panmycin, Tetracap,
    Tetracyn, Robicaps, Robitet)
	Vitamins B3 (niacin), B1 (thiamine), B6 (pyridoxine) and B12 (cobalamin); calcium and magnesium.	

Sulfa Drugs		
Co-Trimoxazole (Septrin) Sulfadiazine Sulfamethoxazole (Gantanol) Trimethoprim (Trimpex, Proloprim, Primsol) Trimethoprim-sulfamethoxazole (Bactrim, Bactrim DS, Septra)	Vitamins B2 (riboflavin), B7 (biotin), B9 (folate), B12 (cobalamin), and K.	
Chloramphenicol (Chloromycetin)	Vitamin B3 (niacin)	
Antifungals		
Fluconazole (Diflucan)	Potassium	
Antituberculosis Drugs		
Cycloserine (Seromycin)	Vitamins B3 (niacin), B9 (folate), and vitamin B6 (pyridoxine); Beneficial gut bacteria.	
Ethambutol (Myambutol)	Copper and zinc. Beneficial gut bacteria.	
Isoniazid (INH)	Vitamins B3 (niacin), vitamin B6 (pyridoxine). Depletes beneficial gut bacteria.	

	Interactions	Notes
		More than 10 days of use is likely to cause vitamin K deficiency.
	Take antibiotic 2 hours before or 4 hours after taking calcium, iron, zinc, or magnesium or consuming dairy products.	
	Take antibiotic 2 hours before or 4 hours after taking calcium, iron, zinc, or magnesium.	
	Take antibiotic 2 hours before or 4 hours after taking vitamins B2 (riboflavin) or B6 (pyridoxine), calcium, iron, zinc, or magnesium.	Do not exceed the UL for vitamin A as it can increase the risk for intercranial hypertension.
		Inhibits the enzyme necessary to make the active form of folate. If taking for more than one month, consider taking 400 mcg of methylfolate and 50 mg of riboflavin per day.
	Do not exceed the DV of vitamin B12. Take antibiotic 2 hours before or 4 hours after taking magnesium.	Consider taking 20 mg per day of vitamin B3.
		Take with food.
		Eat potassium-rich foods. Make sure potassium levels checked if taking for more than 2 months.
	Take drug 2 hours before or 4 hours after taking magnesium.	Inhibits absorption and/or increases metabolism of folate. Blocks conversion of tryptophan to niacin. Inactivates vitamin B6. Levels should be monitored. Consider taking 25–50 mg of P5P, 400 mcg of methylfolate, and 20 mg per day of vitamin B3.
		Decreases absorption of these minerals.
		Interferes with conversion of tryptophan to niacin. Interferes with vitamin B6 metabolism. Levels must be monitored. May increase vitamin D levels. Consider taking 25–50 mg of P5P and 20 mg of vitamin B3 per day.

Drug	Nutrients Depleted	
Pyrazinamide (PZA)	Vitamin B3 (niacin). Beneficial gut bacteria.	
Rifampin (Rifadin, Rofact)	Vitamins D and K. Beneficial gut bacteria.	
Antirheumatics		
Azathioprine (Imuran)	Vitamin B3 (niacin)	
Methotrexate (Rheumatrex, Trexall)	Vitamins B2 (riboflavin), B9 (folic acid), B12 (cobalamin)	
Penicillamine (Cuprimine, Depen)	Copper, iron, magnesium, zinc, vitamin B6 (pyridoxine)	
Cardiovascular Drugs		
ACE Inhibitors		
Benazepril (Lotensin) Captopril (Capoten) Enalapril (Vasotec) Enalapril with hydrochlorothiazide (Vasotec HCT) Fosinopril (Monopril) Lisinopril (Prinivil, Zestril) Moexipril (Univasc) Quinapril (Accupril) Ramipril (Altace, Spirapril) Trandolapril (Mavik)	Zinc	
Enalapril (Vasotec)	CoQ10	
Enalapril with hydrochlorothiazide (Vasotec HCT)	Magnesium, potassium	
Ramipril (Altace)	Potassium	
Alpha 2 Agonists		
Clonidine (Catapres, Duraclon) Methyldopa (Aldomet) Guanfacine (Tenex)	CoQ10	
Angiotensin II Receptor Blockers (ARBs)		
Candesartan with hydrochlorothiazide (Atacand HCT) Irbesartan with hydrochlorothiazide (Avalide) Valsartan (Diovan) Valsartan with hydrochlorothiazide (Diovan HCT)	Zinc	
Antiarrhythmics		
Amiodarone (Cordarone)		

Interactions	Notes
	May interfere with the activity of niacin. Consider taking 20 mg per day of vitamin B3.
	Increases vitamin D metabolism, decreases GI absorption of vitamin K and destroys vitamin K-producing gut bacteria. Must monitor levels; supplements often required.
If taking for cancer, do *not* supplement with folate unless instructed to by an oncologist.	Inhibits conversion to active form of vitamin B3. Consider taking 20 mg of vitamin B3 per day.
	Prevents conversion to active form of folate. Patients taking drug for noncancer conditions should take folate as directed.
	Decreased absorption of minerals. Prevents active form of vitamin B6 in body. Consider taking 25–50 mg of P5P per day.
	Take around mealtime.
Be cautious with salt substitutes, which are often high in potassium chloride. When taken in combination with ACE inhibitors, they can cause a dangerous rise in potassium. Take drug 2 hours before or 4 hours after taking iron supplements.	Increases urinary excretion of zinc. Consider taking 15–25 mg per day of zinc.
	Consider taking 100 mg CoQ10 if over 50.
	Very important to monitor potassium and RBC magnesium levels.
	Potassium must be monitored.
Vitamin B3 (niacin) can intensify effects of this drug. Some authorities caution against high doses (more than 50 mg per day) of vitamin B6 (pyridoxine) because B6 can lower blood pressure further.	If you take more than 35 mg of vitamin B3, take it 4 hours apart from these medications.
Be cautious with salt substitutes, which are often high in potassium chloride. When taken in combination with ARBs, they can cause a dangerous rise in potassium.	May increase urinary excretion of zinc. Consider taking 15–25 mg per day of zinc.
Check with your health-care provider before exceeding DV of vitamin B6. Don't supplement with more than 150 mcg of iodine.	

Drug	Nutrients Depleted	
Beta-Blockers		
Atenolol (Tenormin) Bisoprolol (Zebeta) Esmolol (Brevibloc) Labetalol (Normodyne, Trandate) Metoprolol (Lopressor or Toprol) Nadolol (Corgard) Penbutolol (Levatol) Pindolol (Visken) Propranolol (Inderal) Sotalol (Betapace) Timolol (Betimol, Blocadren, Timoptic)	CoQ10, choline, melatonin, vitamins B1 (thiamine) and D	
Calcium Channel Blockers		
Amlodipine (Norvasc) Bepridil (Vascor) Diltiazem (Cardizem, Dilacor) Felodipine (Plendil) Nifedipine (Procardia) Verapamil (Calan, Isoptin)	Melatonin, vitamin D	
Cardiac Glycosides		
Digoxin (Lanoxin, Lanoxicaps, Digibind)	Vitamin B1 (thiamine), magnesium	
Diuretics, Loop		
Bumetanide (Bumex) Ethacrynic acid (Edecrin) Furosemide (Lasix) Torsemide (Demadex)	Vitamins B1 (thiamine), B6 (pyridoxine), B9 (folate) and C; calcium, magnesium, potassium, sodium, zinc	
Diuretics, Potassium-Sparing		
Amiloride (Midamor) Hydrochlorothiazide and triamterene (Dyazide, Maxzide) Spironolactone (Aldactone) Triamterene (Dyrenium)	Calcium, vitamin B9 (folate)	
Diuretics, Thiazide		
Chlorothiazide (Diuril) Hydrochlorothiazide (Aquazide, Esidrix, Ezide, Hydrocot, HydroDIURIL, Mirozide) Indapamide (Lozol) Methyclothiazide (Aquatensen, Enduron) Metolazone (Mykrox, Zaroxolyn)	Vitamins B1 (thiamine), B2 (riboflavin), and B9 (folate); CoQ10, magnesium, potassium, sodium, zinc	
Vasodilator		
Hydralazine (Apresoline)	Vitamin B6 (pyridoxine), magnesium, CoQ10	
Chemotherapy Drugs		
There are many drugs used to treat cancer.	Many nutrients are depleted. These are specific to the chemotherapy drug being used.	

Interactions	Notes
Do not drink orange juice within 2 hours of taking atenolol (reduces drug's effectiveness). Vitamin E supplements may interfere with absorption of these drugs. Take 4 hours apart. Monitor blood pressure if taking more than 50 mg of vitamin B6. Do not exceed the DV of calcium from *all* sources.	These drugs block the production of melatonin and CoQ10. Consider taking 3 mg melatonin and 100–200 mg of CoQ10 per day.
Do not exceed the DV of calcium or magnesium without taking to your health-care provider.	Can reduce synthesis of vitamin D. Check calcium and vitamin D levels *before* supplementing with more than the DV of either and monitor periodically. Consider taking 3 mg of melatonin if having insomnia.
Do not exceed the DV of calcium or vitamin D without talking to your health-care provider. Do not take magnesium within 4 hours of drug. Do not take St. John's wort.	Monitor B1 and RBC magnesium levels. Deficiency can be dangerous. Supplements often necessary.
	Monitor vitamins B1 and B6, potassium, sodium, and RBC magnesium levels closely. Nutrient deficiencies common. Supplements almost always necessary.
Be cautious with salt substitutes, which are often high in potassium chloride. When taken in combination with ARBs, they can cause a dangerous rise in potassium.	Amiloride can elevate zinc levels. Do not exceed the DV for zinc without talking to your health-care provider.
Do not exceed 1,000 IU per day vitamin D3 or the DV of calcium from *all sources* without talking to your health-care provider.	Monitor vitamin B1, potassium, and RBC magnesium levels closely. Consider taking a B-complex, 15–25 mg of zinc, and 300 mg per day of magnesium.
	Monitor blood pressure if taking more than 50 mg per day of vitamin B6.
While nutrient support is important, certain nutrients may reduce the effectiveness of specific drugs.	You must talk to an integrative oncologist or dietitian to determine what supplements you should and should not take during treatment.

Drug	Nutrients Depleted	
Cholesterol-Lowering Drugs		
Bile Acid Sequestrants		
Cholestyramine (Questran) Colestipol (Colestid) Colesevelam (Welchol)	Vitamins A, B9 (folate), B12 (cobalamin), D, E, and K; calcium, magnesium, and iron.	
Fibric Acid Derivatives		
Gemfibrozil (Lopid)	Vitamin E, CoQ10	
Statins		
Atorvastatin (Lipitor) Fluvastatin (Lescol) Lovastatin (Mevacor) Pravastatin (Pravachol) Simvastatin (Zocor)	CoQ10	
Dermatology Drugs		
Calcipotriene (Dovonex)		
Isotretinoin (Accutane, Claravis, Isotrex) Acitretin (Soriatane)	Acetyl-l-carnitine	
Diabetes Drugs		
Biguanide		
Metformin (Glucophage, Glucophage XR, Glumetza, Fortamet)	Vitamins B1 (thiamine), B9 (folate), and B12 (coabalamin); possibly CoQ10	
Sulfonylurea		
Acetohexamide (Dymelor) Chlorpropamide (Diabinese) Glipizide (Glucotrol) Glyburide (Diabeta, Glynase, Micronase) Tolazamide (Tolinase) Tolbutamide (Orinase, Tol-Tab)	CoQ10	
Insulin		
Short, rapid, and long-acting insulin, as well as premixed	Magnesium	
Estrogen/ Hormone Therapy		
Conjugated estrogens (Premarin) Conjugated estrogens, synthetic (Cenestin, Enjuvia) Esterified estrogens (Estratab, Menest) Estradiol (Estrace, Estraderm, Alora, Climara, FemPatch, Vivelle) Estropipate (Ogen)	*Vitamins A, B1 (thiamine), B2 (riboflavin), B6 (pyridoxine), B12 (cobalamin), and C; magnesium, zinc*	

Interactions	Notes
Take drug at least 2 hours before or 4 hours after taking nutritional supplements.	Reduces the absorption of fat-soluble vitamins, as well as key minerals. Multivitamin-mineral strongly recommended.
	Mechanism of nutrient depletion is not known. Consider taking 100–200 mg of CoQ10.
Do not drink grapefruit juice; it will cause statin levels to rise, which can be dangerous to the liver and muscles. High doses of vitamin D may reduce the effectiveness of atorvastatin.	Statin drugs block the synthesis of mevalonic acid, which is a precursor of CoQ10. Consider taking 100–200 mg/d of CoQ10. Do *not* take red yeast rice if taking statins.
Supplement only the beta-carotene form of vitamin A (i.e., avoid retinol supplements).	Drug is a synthetic vitamin D. Ask your health-care provider to monitor calcium and vitamin D levels *before* exceeding the DV of calcium or vitamin D. Consider supplementing with 1,000 mg per day of acetyl-l-carnitine.
Monitor blood sugar if taking chromium, alpha-lipoic acid or other nutrients that might lower blood sugar. Adjust medication if needed.	Calcium may reduce vitamin B12 depletion. Vitamin B12 levels should be checked annually. Consider taking 500 mcg per day of vitamin B12, 600 mg 1–2 times per day of alpha-lipoic acid, and a multivitamin-mineral.
Monitor blood sugar if taking chromium, alpha-lipoic acid or other nutrients that might lower blood sugar. Adjust medication if needed.	Long-term use depletes CoQ10. Consider taking 100–200 mg per day of CoQ10.
Monitor blood sugar if taking chromium, alpha-lipoic acid, or other nutrients that might lower blood sugar. Adjust medication if needed.	Increases urinary excretion of magnesium. RBC magnesium levels should be monitored. Consider taking 300–400 mg per day of magnesium.
	Women taking estrogen therapy for menopause should take a multivitamin-mineral.

Drug	Nutrients Depleted	
Gastrointestinal Drugs		
Antacids and Acid Blockers		
Antacids		
Aluminum and magnesium hydroxide (Gaviscon, Mylanta, Maalox) Calcium carbonate (Rolaids, Tums) Magnesium hydroxide (Milk of Magnesia) Sodium bicarbonate (Alka-Seltzer, baking soda)	Vitamins B7 (biotin), and B9 (folate); calcium, chromium, iron, CoQ10	
H2 Blockers		
Cimetidine (Tagamet) Famotidine (Pepcid) Nizatidine (Axid) Ranitidine (Zantac, Taladine)	Vitamins B7 (biotin) and B9 (folate); calcium, iron, zinc, melatonin, CoQ10	
Proton-Pump Inhibitors		
Esomeprazole (Nexium) Lansoprazole (Prevacid) Omeprazole (Prilosec, Zegerid) Pantoprazole (Protonix) Rabeprazole (Aciphex)	Vitamins A, B1 (thiamine), B2 (riboflavin) B6 (pyridoxine) B7 (biotin), B9 (folate) B12 (cobalamin), C, and D; calcium, chromium, iron, magnesium, selenium, melatonin, CoQ10	
GI Anti-inflammatory		
Sulfasalazine (Azulfidine)	Vitamins B6 (pyridoxine), B9 (folate) and B12 (cobalamin)	
Gout Drugs		
Colchicine	Vitamins B9 (folate), B12 (cobalamin), and D; beta-carotene, magnesium, potassium	
Probenacid	Vitamin B2 (riboflavin)	
Mental Health Drugs		
Antianxiety Drugs		
Alprazolam (Xanax) Clonazepam (Klonopin) Diazepam (Valium) Lorazepam (Ativan)	Melatonin	
Antidepressants		
Monoamine Oxidase Inhibitors		
Isocarboxazid (Marplan) Phenelzine (Nardil) Rasagiline (Azilect) Tranylcypromine (Parnate) Selegiline (Emsam)	Vitamin B6 (pyridoxine)	
Serotonin Reuptake Inhibitors		
Citalopram (Celexa) Escitalopram (Lexapro) Fluoxetine (Prozac, Sarafem) Sertraline (Zoloft) Paroxetine (Paxil)	Melatonin, iodine, selenium, vitamin B9 (folate)	

Interactions	Notes
	All deplete the body of beneficial bacteria. Take a high quality probiotic blend of Lactobacillus and Bifidobacteria
Vitamin C can increase absorption of aluminum in antacids. Do not exceed 500 mg per day of vitamin C.	Folate deficiency likely if taking large doses for more than 1 year. Non-heme iron and chromium absorption are reduced. Monitor levels.
If taking calcium, use noncarbonate form (e.g., citrate).	Risk for B12 deficiency increases if taking high doses for more than one year and over age 50. Monitor level annually. Consider taking 500 mcg per day of vitamin B12.
If taking calcium, use noncarbonate form (e.g., citrate). Cranberry juice may enhance absorption of vitamin B12.	Risk for magnesium and B12 deficiency if taken for more than one year and over age 50. Non-heme iron is not well absorbed. Vitamin C destroyed at higher pH. Fracture risk elevated. Consider taking 500 mcg of vitamin B12, 200 mg of vitamin C twice daily, 2,000 IU of vitamin D, and 300–400 mg of magnesium.
Take probiotic and iron supplements 4 hours after medication.	Drug is best taken after a meal. Folate is almost always necessary. Level should be monitored.
	Drug blocks conversion of beta-carotene to vitamin A. Use multiple vitamin containing preformed vitamin A.
	Decreased absorption and enhanced urinary excretion. Consider taking 50–100 mg per day of vitamin B2.
	Take with or without food.
	Consider taking 1–3 mg of melatonin 2 hours before bedtime.
	Significant food interactions.
Do not take St. John's Wort, 5-HTP or SAMe with these drugs.	*Many* foods to avoid: cheese, cured meats, fava beans, beer, wine, and sauerkraut, yogurt, bananas, and avocados, to name just a few. Monitor vitamin B6 levels closely.
	Take with food or snack.
Do not take St. John's wort, 5-HTP, or SAMe without talking to your health-care provider first.	Consider taking 1–3 mg of melatonin 2 hours before bedtime and multivitamin-mineral.

Drug	Nutrients Depleted	
Serotonin-Norepinephrine Reuptake Inhibitors		
Desvenlafaxine (Pristiq) Duloxetine (Cymbalta) Venlafaxine (Effexor)	Possibly vitamin B12 (cobalamin)	
Tricylic Antidepressants		
Amitriptyline (Elavil) Clomipramine (Anafranil) Desipramine (Norpramin) Doxepin (Sinequan) Imipramine (Tofranil) Nortriptyline (Aventyl, Pamelor) Protriptyline (Vivactil)	CoQ10, vitamin B2 (riboflavin)	
Others		
Bupropion (Wellbutrin) Mirtazapine (Remeron)	Vitamin B6 (pyridoxine), vitamin C vitamin D, CoQ10	
Antipsychotics		
Chlorpromazine (Thorazine) Fluphenazine (Permitil, Prolixin) Haloperidol (Haldol) Mesoridazine (Serentil) Perphenazine (Trilafon) Prochlorperazine (Compazine) Thioridazine (Mellaril) Thiothixene (Navane) Trifluoperazine (Stelazine)	CoQ10, melatonin, vitamin B2 (riboflavin)	
Others		
Lithium	Vitamin B9 (folate) and inositol	
Olanzapine (Zyprexa) Quetiapine (Seroquel) Risperidone (Risperdal)	Vitamins A, B1(thiamine), B7 (biotin), B9 (folate), B12 (cobalamin), C, D and K; calcium, and carnitine	
Oral Contraceptives		
All monophasic, biphasic and triphasic preparations	Vitamins B2 (riboflavin), B5 (pantothenic acid), B6 (pyridoxine) B9 (folate), B12 (cobalamin), vitamin C, magnesium, and zinc	
Osteoporosis drugs		
Bisphosphonates		
Alendronate (Fosamax) Risedronate (Actonel) Etidronate (Didronel) Ibandronate (Boniva) Pamidronate (Aredia) Tiludronate (Skelid) Zoledronic acid (Reclast, Zometa)	Calcium	

Interactions	Notes
	Take with food or snack.
Do not take St. John's wort, 5-HTP, or SAMe without talking to your health-care provider first.	Consider taking multivitamin-mineral.
	Take with food or snack.
Vitamin E supplements may interfere with absorption of these drugs. Take 4 hours apart. Do not take St. John's wort, 5-HTP, or SAMe without talking to your health-care provider first.	These drugs deplete riboflavin. Taking vitamins B2 and/or B6 may improve the drug's effectiveness. Consider taking 50–100 mg of vitamin B2, 25–50 mg of P5P, and 100–200 mg CoQ10.
Do not take St. John's wort, 5-HTP, or SAMe without talking to your health-care provider first.	Can take with food or empty stomach. Consider taking multivitamin/mineral.
	Usually on empty stomach. Take with food if stomach upset.
Vitamin E supplements may interfere with absorption of these drugs. Take 4 hours apart.	Melatonin may help reduce the risk of tardive dyskinesia, an often irreversible condition caused by these drugs. Consider taking 3–5 melatonin 2 hours before bedtime, 100–200 mg of CoQ10, and 50–100 mg of vitamin B2.
Do not take more than 150 mcg of supplemental potassium iodide. Lithium should be taken after a meal to decrease side effects and blood levels of the drug regularly monitored.	Lithium decreases excretion of calcium. Do not exceed the daily value from all sources for calcium. Consider taking 1,000 mg per day of inositol. Monitor folate levels. Take a high-quality multivitamin-mineral with adequate vitamin B-complex. Maintain vitamin D level >30 ng/mL.
	Take with food.
Do not regularly drink grapefruit juice, as it can increase estrogen levels by up to 30 percent.	Oral contraceptives may increase vitamin A levels in the body. Do not exceed 3,000 IU of preformed vitamin A. Oral contraceptives increase iron levels; do not exceed the DV of iron. Women should take a good multivitamin/mineral.
	Take on empty stomach.
Do not take calcium, iron, magnesium, or trace minerals within 2 hours of taking your medication.	Ensure you are meeting daily value for calcium and have vitamin D levels monitored to keep level >30 ng/mL.

Drug	Nutrients Depleted		
Parkinson's Drugs			
Levodopa (Dopar, Larodopa) Levodopa-carbidopa (Sinimet, Rytary, Duopa) Levodopa-carbidopa-entacapone (Stalevo)	Vitamin B3 (niacin)		
Respiratory Drugs			
Beta 2 Agonists			
Albuterol (Proventil, Ventolin) Bitolterol (Tornalate) Levalbuterol (Xopenex) Metaproterenol (Alupent) Pirbuterol (Maxair) Salmeterol (Serevent) Terbutaline (Brethaire)	Magnesium, potassium		
Inhaled Corticosteroids			
Beclomethasone (Qvar) Budesonide (Pulmicort) Flunisolide (Aerobid) Fluticasone (Flovent) Triamcinolone (Azmacort)	Vitamins A, B6 (pyridoxine), B9 (folate), B12 (cobalamin) and D; calcium, magnesium, melatonin, selenium, and zinc		
Leukotriene Modifiers			
Montelukast (Singulair) Zafirlukast (Accolate)	Possibly essential fatty acids and potassium.		
Methylxanthines			
Theophylline (Slo-Bid, Theo-Dur, Theo-24, Theolair) Aminophylline Oxtriphylline (Choledyl SA) Dyphylline (Lufyllin) Dextromethorphan (Robitussin DM)	Vitamin B6 (pyridoxine), potassium		
Steroid Drugs			
Prednisone Prednisolone Methylprednisolone Hydrocortisone	Vitamins B6 (pyridoxine), B9 (folic acid), C, D, and K; calcium, chromium, magnesium, potassium, selenium, zinc		
Thyroid Drugs			
Levothyroxine (Levothroid, Synthroid Unithroid) Armour thyroid Liothyronine (Cytomel) Compounded products	Calcium		
Weight-Loss Drugs			
Orlistat (Alli, Xenical)	Vitamins A, D, E, and K		

Interactions	Notes
	Usually taken 15–30 minutes before meal.
Do not take iron within 4 hours of taking medication. Do not take SAMe when on taking any of these drugs.	Do not take vitamin B6 if taking levodopa as a single drug. Taking the DV of vitamin B6 is not an issue if taking levodopa in combination with carbidopa. Monitor vitamin B3 levels.
	Take with or without food.
	Electrolyte levels should be closely monitored. Consider taking 300–400 mg per day of magnesium and eat potassium-rich foods.
	Take with or without food.
	Inhaled corticosteroids have fewer risks of nutrient depletion than systemic. Ensure adequate calcium and vitamin D level >30 ng/mL. Take a high-quality multivitamin-mineral.
	Take with or without food.
	Consider supplementing with omega-3 fatty acids. Eat potassium-rich foods.
	Best taken on empty stomach. Take with food if upsets stomach.
	Inhibits conversion to active form of vitamin B6. Consider taking 25–50 mg per day of P5P. Eat diet rich in potassium foods and have levels monitored.
Do not take SAMe while taking dextromethorphan	
	Take with food.
Ensure adequate protein intake.	Roughly 1 in 5 cases of osteoporosis due to long-term use of corticosteroids. Keep vitamin D levels >30 ng/mL; consider increasing calcium to 1,300 mg per day from all sources. Chromium may protect against steroid-induced diabetes.
	Take thyroid on an empty stomach.
Take drug 2 hours before or 4 hours after taking iron, alpha-lipoic acid, magnesium, calcium or consuming dairy supplements. Vitamin C enhances	Calcium loss only a problem if taking high doses of thyroid hormones. Do not exceed 150 mcg of supplemental potassium iodide. Vitamin C enhances absorption of thyroid medication.
	Take with meal or within one hour after meal.
	The absorption of all fat-soluble vitamins is impaired. Consider taking high-quality multivitamin-mineral and maintain vitamin D levels >30 ng/mL.

Glossary

antioxidants—Agents known to prevent oxidative stress, an imbalance at the cellular level that leads to DNA damage that can cause aging, illness, and disease.

bioflavonoids—Antioxidant compounds found in some fruits and vegetables, particularly citrus fruits and green tea.

blood-brain barrier—A biological gate that prevents many substances in the bloodstream from entering the brain, thereby protecting it from potential damage from toxins.

botanical medicine—Another term for herbal medicine, which employs the use of plants for the treatment of illness and/or promotion of health. Botanical or herbal remedies can be used as teas; taken as capsules, liquids, or tablets; or applied topically to skin.

free radicals—Molecules with an unpaired electron, making them highly reactive.

heme—Iron-containing compound found in hemoglobin.

hemoglobin—Protein molecule in red blood cells that contains iron and is responsible for transporting oxygen. *See:* heme.

longitudinal study—Studies based on the observation of large numbers of people over a long period of time. Examples include the Framingham Heart Study, the Health Professionals Study, and the Nurses' Health Study.

low-glycemic load foods—Foods that do not cause a dramatic or rapid rise in one's blood sugar level after consumption. Examples include tomatoes, apples, lettuce, and whole wheat bread.

Mediterranean diet—Traditional dietary pattern of people living around the Mediterranean sea, featuring abundant fresh vegetables and fruit, beans, nuts, whole grains, fish, olive oil, and modest amounts of meat, cheese, and red wine.

megaloblastic anemia—A form of anemia characterized by large, immature red blood cells that is often the result of a vitamin B9 and/or B12 deficiency.

meta-analysis—A study that analyzes multiple data points and statistics from other studies to draw its conclusions. While not infallible, meta-analysis can be an incredibly helpful tool for making evidence based recommendations in medicine.

mitochondria—The power centers in our cells, where respiration and the production of energy occur.

nutraceutical—While there is no legal or regulatory definition of nutraceuticals, the term is used in the supplement industry to describe all the nutritional supplements that do not fit neatly into the strict categories of vitamins, minerals, essential fatty acids, or botanical/herbal supplements. Examples include glucosamine, chondroitin, or SAMe.

oxidative stress—Oxidation is simply the removal of electrons from an atom or a molecule. Electrons like to travel in pairs, and when one is removed it becomes a free radical that is capable of damaging body tissues. Oxidative stress is the total burden on the body caused by the constant production of these free radicals. Keeping the body supplied with dietary antioxidants helps reduce this burden.

phytonutrients—*Phyto* in Greek means "plant," hence these are nutrients found in plants that are not strictly vitamins, minerals, fats, carbohydrates, or proteins. Examples include quercetin, anthocyanins, and resveratrol.

prebiotics—Dietary fiber that promotes development of a healthy population of microorganism in the digestive system.

precursor—Any substance that is transformed into another. It often refers to an inactive substance that is transformed to an active one.

prediabetes—When blood sugar and insulin levels are elevated but not enough to qualify for the diagnosis of diabetes.

vegan—A person who does not eat any animal products, including meat, dairy, eggs, or fish.

vegetarian—A person who does not eat meat. Vegetarians may be lacto (abstain from all meat and eggs but eat dairy), lacto-ovo (abstain from meat but consume eggs and dairy products), or pescatarian (avoid all meat but include fish), though this latter category is not by strict definition vegetarian.

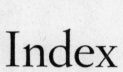

Index

About the Author

Tieraona Low Dog, M.D., is an internationally recognized expert in the fields of dietary supplements, herbal medicine, women's health, and natural medicine. Her career in natural medicine began more than 35 years ago. She studied midwifery, massage therapy, martial arts, and was a highly respected herbalist, serving as president of the American Herbalist Guild before going on to receive her doctor of medicine degree from the University of New Mexico School of Medicine. She currently serves as the fellowship director for the Academy of Integrative Health and Medicine, where she leads the nation's first interprofessional graduate level training program in integrative medicine.

In addition to her work as a clinician and educator, Dr. Low Dog has been involved in national health policy and regulatory issues for more than fifteen years. In 2000, she was appointed by President Bill Clinton to serve on the White House Commission of Complementary and Alternative Medicine and then served on the advisory council for the National Institutes of Health National Center for Complementary and Integrative Health. She was the elected chair of the United States Pharmacopeia Dietary

Supplements–Botanicals Expert Committee from 2000 to 2010 and the elected chair of the U.S. Pharmacopeia Dietary Supplements Admission Evaluation Committee from 2010 to 2015. She is a founding member of the American Board of Physician Specialties American Board of Integrative Medicine and the Academy of Women's Health.

An invited speaker at more than 550 scientific/medical conferences and a frequent guest on *The Dr. Oz Show* and NPR's *The People's Pharmacy,* Dr. Low Dog has published 45 peer-reviewed articles, written 22 chapters for medical textbooks, and published 5 books, including National Geographic's *Life Is Your Best Medicine* and *Healthy at Home.* She co-authored the *National Geographic Guide to Medicinal Herbs* and was co-editor of *Integrative Women's Health* by Oxford University Press. Named by *Time* magazine as an "innovator in complementary and alternative medicine" (2001), she also received the Burton Kallman Scientific Award (2007), the People's Pharmacy Award for Excellence in Research and Communication for the Public Health (2010), the New York Zen Center's Contemplative Care Award (2013), the Integrative Healthcare Leadership Award (2014), and the American Herbal Products Association's Herbal Insight Award (2015).

Ad TK